The Sainsbury Book of

First Aid

Brian Ward
Consultant: Dr P F Green
MB ChB (Edin)

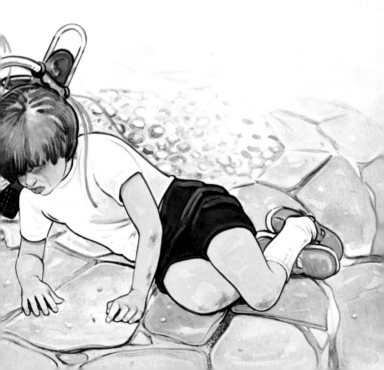

Contents

Published exclusively for J Sainsbury Limited
Stamford Street, London SE1 9LL
by Cathay Books
59 Grosvenor Street, London W1

First published 1981

© Cathay Books 1981
ISBN 0 86178 071 X

Printed in Hong Kong

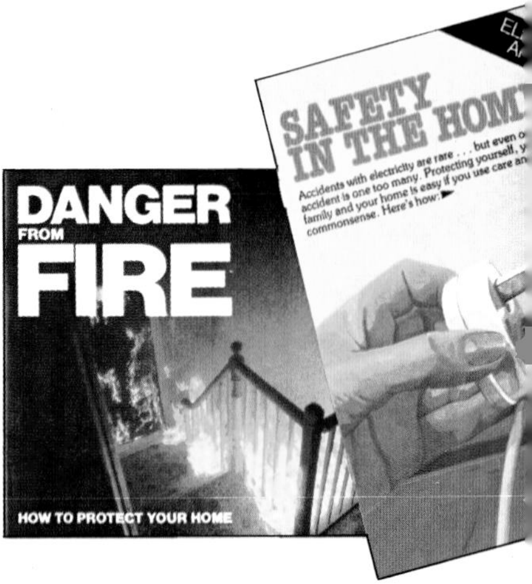

Some of the many
leaflets designed
to promote safety
in the home

DANGER FROM FIRE

SAFETY IN THE HOME

HOW TO PROTECT YOUR HOME

Introduction

With a few rare exceptions, accidents are caused by people – not by the inanimate objects which actually inflict the damage – and common sense can prevent most of them.

Legislation protects us from major hazards. Standards and regulations control home construction, electricity and gas supply, motoring and other forms of transport, and most other obvious potential causes of serious accidents. But it is not possible to legislate against the minor accidents caused by carelessness or forgetfulness.

Electricity and gas are obvious hazards about the home, and most adults have a healthy respect for them. Children do not, and they need protecting from themselves. So do the elderly, who may become forgetful or careless. Even the most generally careful of us are forgetful on occasion. If we wake up and go downstairs in the night, for example, we are not usually fully alert. Similarly, illnesses such as influenza can leave us physically weak and light-headed.

Then, everyday objects seem to take on a life of their own. A kitchen knife inevitably falls point-first when it is dropped on your foot; the careless match is struck before the gas leak is noticed.

There is no way, short of living in a padded cell, in which you can prevent every hazard. But you can take a long, hard look at your home, your work, and your leisure, and try to anticipate how your environment and these everyday activities could turn against you.

To help you, on the following pages we draw attention to potential hazards, suggest ways of avoiding them and advise you how to cope in an emergency. (Please note that medical ethics preclude the author and consultant from entering into correspondence with individual members of the public.)

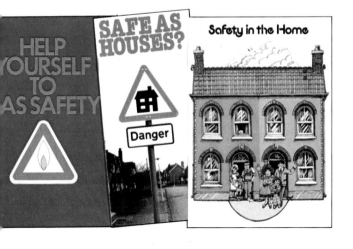

1: Commonsense and Accident Prevention

General domestic hazards

Are you sitting comfortably reading this book in the safety of your own home? If you are, don't be too complacent. There is as much risk of a fatal accident in your own home as there is out on the roads.

As a result of accidents occurring in the home, every day in Britain 18 people die, and each year 1½ million people need hospital treatment. The worst domestic hazards to adults are falls (mostly affecting the elderly), burns, and cuts. Children are especially at risk from burns, poisoning and suffocation.

Falls are probably the most dangerous, and they almost always result from a momentary lapse in attention. Rushing downstairs to answer the telephone or door bell perhaps, you slip, or trip over some unnoticed obstacle like a toy, and a sprained ankle may be the least serious injury sustained.

Uncarpeted stair treads are slippery, and therefore dangerous, while the risks from badly fitted or torn stair carpet are obvious.

Just tripping over a badly laid floor carpet can cause a nasty fall, so

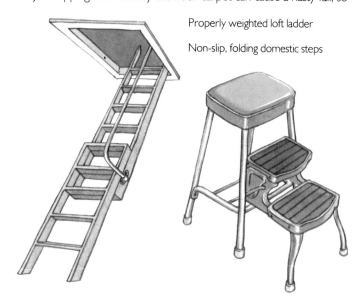

Properly weighted loft ladder

Non-slip, folding domestic steps

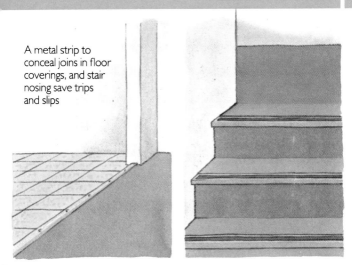

A metal strip to conceal joins in floor coverings, and stair nosing save trips and slips

make sure that all floor covering is fixed down securely. Joins in floor covering are a particular hazard, especially in doorways where they should be covered with one of the proprietary metal strips designed for this purpose. Loose mats are even more dangerous. You can trip, or skid on them if they are laid on a shiny floor – never polish under your mats or rugs. Better still, fit non-slip grips.

Risks are reduced if you can see the hazards. Always switch lights on before going downstairs at night, and make sure that lighting throughout the home is adequate. The cost of putting more powerful light bulbs in hallways and passages is only a few pence per year, and if only a bruise or sprained ankle is avoided, you can consider the money well spent.

Most people tend to store seldom-used items high up, out of reach. Climbing on a chair is only safe if the item you are reaching for is then within easy grasp, and if the chair is securely positioned so that it cannot tip. But it is much safer to use a small set of folding domestic steps that allow you to reach even the highest cupboard easily. Always fold the steps safely away immediately after use. This is, of course, particularly important if you have young children and the high cupboards are sited above busy, potentially dangerous worktops, as in the kitchen shelf shown overleaf.

Attic access is especially dangerous without a fixed staircase, and a properly weighted loft ladder is the only sensible alternative. A slip from a precariously balanced chair beneath an attic trapdoor means a fall of 2 m (7 ft) or more, and it may mean falling over the banisters and on to the staircase.

In the attic, have you boarded across the joists to make it safe to walk about? If not, you stand a good chance of putting a foot through the ceiling below, or injuring yourself badly by falling right through.

The special problems of domestic safety for children are considered on pages 24–27, and for the elderly on pages 28–29.

Safety in the kitchen

No part of the home is potentially more dangerous than the kitchen. Think of all the hazards present here. Sharp knives, naked flames or hotplates, water and electrical appliances (always a dangerous combination), boiling water and hot irons. Above all, yourself, surrounded by all these dangerous objects.

The kitchen is the busiest room in the home, often used for eating, ironing, and a host of other activities. If there are young children in the household, they will spend much of their time in the kitchen, providing added distraction and hazard.

Kitchen safety begins with a well-planned overall layout and

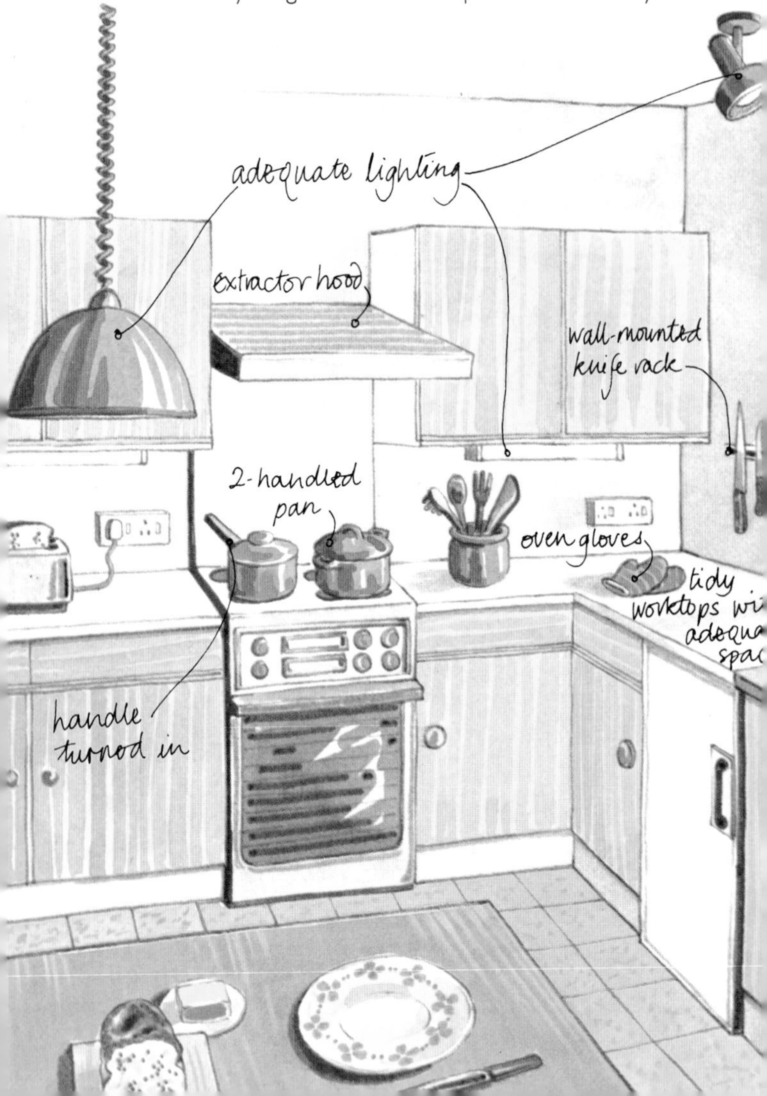

adequate lighting

extractor hood

wall-mounted knife rack

2-handled pan

oven gloves

tidy worktops wi adequa spac

handle turned in

adequate working surfaces at a proper height to allow you to be methodical in your work, automatically reducing the chance of accidents. If you work surrounded by a clutter of utensils, it is easy to drop something on the floor or on your foot, or cut yourself while rummaging about for a mislaid knife.

Wipe up spilt food or liquids right away. Most kitchens have smooth vinyl or composition floors which are extremely slippery when wet or greasy. When planning or redecorating your kitchen, choose a floor covering with a non-slip surface, and one that is easily washable and impervious to water. It will dry quickly and remain cleaner and more hygienic than porous materials, such as carpet or untreated cork tiles.

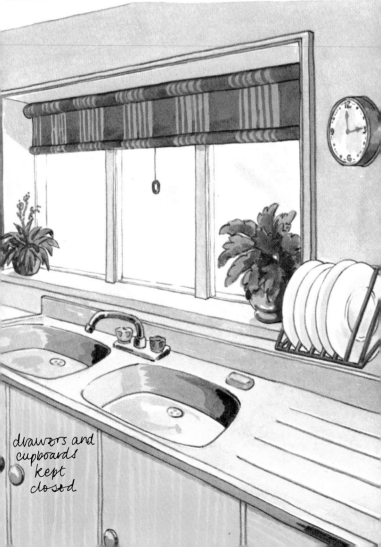

drawers and cupboards kept closed

Burns and scalds

Cooking is the most frequent cause of accidents in the kitchen, where burns and scalds can happen only too easily. Safeguard yourself against splashes and spits from hot oil or fat, or boiling water by wearing a fabric reinforced plastic apron that will not allow hot liquids to penetrate and be held against your skin.

Disposal of hot fat or oil can be very risky. **Never**, ever, run water into hot fat or oil, the temperature of which will probably be much higher than the boiling point of water, so the result will be a blinding, scalding cloud of steam, possibly causing you to suffer terrible burns.

Always try to let fat or oil cool in the pan, before attempting disposal. If you must get rid of it quickly, tip it into a thick wad of old newspaper – *not* down the sink, where it will immediately congeal and produce a total blockage.

Get into the habit of using oven gloves or an oven cloth, kept in a conspicuous spot conveniently near the cooker. If you use gloves or a cloth as a matter of routine you are much less likely to pick up a hot dish absent-mindedly with the risk of painful burns.

Kitchen burns or scalds are often caused by lifting pan lids so that steam shoots out towards you. Always lift the far side of the lid first, and let the steam disperse before looking into the pot. **Never** lean across one hot pan to look in another on the far side of the hob.

If you have weak wrists it is often safer to use pans with small handles on either side, which need both hands to pick them up, rather than the usual type with a single handle. A two-handed grip is more secure, and the pan is less likely to be knocked off the top of the cooker if you catch it accidentally. If you do have pans with single handles, turn them so that the handles do not jut out over the edge of the stove where they can be easily knocked. This is particularly important if you have small children.

Cuts

Very sharp kitchen knives are among the most dangerous items in the home, and should be treated with respect. Never drop them carelessly into a drawer full of other utensils. To eliminate the risk of picking them up by the blade, store them in a wall-mounted knife-rack, above the working surface. They will stay sharper, too.

Be conscious of the damage a large knife can do: carry it pointed away from you as you move about the kitchen and don't carry it about unnecessarily. Cut food on a proper chopping board, and always make the cutting movement away from you, with your fingers well tucked in, away from the blade.

Another frequent cause of cuts is the ordinary tin opener, and the opened tin. Some tin openers have a spike which must be forced into the lid of the tin, which can easily tip over as pressure is applied, neatly spiking your hand. The practice of part-opening the lid is also

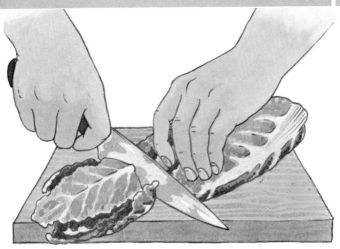

Keep fingers well tucked in when using a sharp knife

hazardous, as the jagged cut edges of both tin and lid are extremely sharp and fingers and knuckles are liable to be cut or trapped while removing food. It is better to take the lid right off, and throw it away.

Clean your can opener thoroughly after each use. Food deposits on the cutter can grow a horrifying assortment of bacteria.

Poisoning

Another major hazard in the kitchen is poisoning. The average kitchen contains many poisonous solutions: bleaches, polishes, oven cleaner, medicines, and so on. Absolutely everything of this nature should be kept well out of children's reach. It is common sense to keep any poison or suspect materials out of the food cupboard, to avoid absent-minded accidents or possible spillages.

The worst risk of poisoning comes from food itself. Always read the instructions on prepacked foods carefully, and pay particular attention to shelf life or "use-by" dates. Be careful not to let fresh meat drip onto cooked foods in the fridge.

The dangers of reheating cooked foods are well known, as food poisoning is a common hazard. Of equal importance are careful defrosting of frozen meat and especially of frozen poultry.

Don't neglect the kitchen waste bin. Wrap waste food in paper before discarding it, to prevent food splashes around the bin which could encourage bacteria and disease-carrying flies. Clean and disinfect the waste bin each time it is emptied, and use plastic bin liners for extra hygiene and convenience.

Bleach is another kitchen hazard, because it is frequently misused. If you pour bleach down the sink waste-pipe to disinfect and clean it, pour carefully. Undiluted bleach splashed onto the skin, and especially onto the face, can produce severe burns or even blindness.

Electricity in the home

Properly fitted and properly used electrical appliances should be 100 per cent safe. There are very stringent codes of practice laid down for electrical installations and appliances, and these are designed to ensure your safety. Accidents are usually the result of damage, incorrect use, or unskilled attempts at repairs.

Wiring up appliances

Your first contact with safety measures comes in connecting up the appliance. Most homes built or rewired after 1947 have 13 amp ring circuit systems. These are more convenient than the old type because each plug now has its own fuse, which will "blow" and break the circuit in the event of an electrical fault. In this system, plugs have 3 rectangular-sectioned pins. When buying plugs, look for the British Standards code BS 1363, and if they will be used where there is any possibility of them taking the occasional knock (near a workbench perhaps) "Smashproof" plugs or Tough-plugs are available. Super safety plugs, designed to be "childproof" are also available.

All BS 1363 13 amp plugs are supplied with detailed wiring instructions which must be followed to the letter. All domestic appliances made since 1970 are already fitted with a colour-coded flexible cable, with its three wires coloured brown for Live, blue for Neutral, and green/yellow for Earth. Flexes on older appliances, and the cable built into the house wiring, are coloured red for Live; black for Neutral; green for Earth. If no details come with the plug, look for tiny code letters printed or moulded into the plug, near each pin: L for Live, N for Neutral, E or ⏚ for Earth.

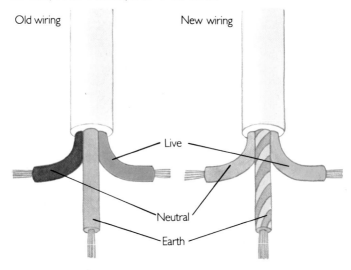

Old wiring   New wiring

Live

Neutral

Earth

Some appliances carry a label marked: "Double Insulated". These are specially designed to be safe without an earth connection, so for these appliances *only*, the two leads are connected to the Live and Neutral terminals – the Earth pin in the plug is left unconnected.

When preparing the flex, first cut away 5 cm (2 in) of the outer sheath, then strip off about 1 cm (½ in) of plastic insulation from the end of each conducting wire, by cutting round it with a sharp knife or special stripping tool. Be careful not to cut the copper conductor. Then pull off the short piece of plastic sleeve. Twist the exposed strands of each wire together to make a smooth bundle with no stray strands. This is normally inserted into a hole in the terminal pin, and clamped down tightly with a screw. If there are no holes in the pins, the exposed twists of wire are looped *clockwise* round their respective terminals and clamped beneath a special nut and washer.

The flex leads out through a gap at one end of the plug, underneath a clamp which must firmly grip the sheath of the flex to stop the thin conductor wires being pulled out of the terminals. Then screw the plug together.

NB Always follow installation instructions provided with the plug as these may vary in detail between different makes. If in any doubt get expert advice before proceeding.

Fuses and fuse ratings
Fuses are fitted in the plug for its protection and that of the flex. They allow the safe amount of power to pass through to an appliance, but "blow" if overloading or insulation failure occurs. The modern 13 amp plug is usually supplied fitted with a 13 amp fuse, which is adequate to cope with most portable domestic appliance

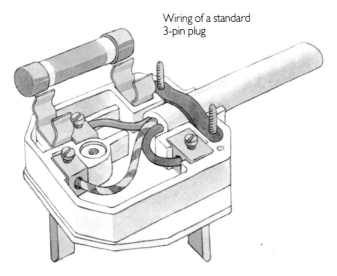

Wiring of a standard
3-pin plug

3 amp fuses are suitable for
most appliances up to 700 watts

13 amp fuses are
suitable for appliances of 700
to 3000 watts

Typical wired fuse

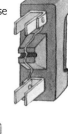

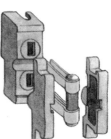

Cartridge fuse

loadings. But in some cases, a much smaller fuse rating is needed. The instructions with the appliance will specify the required fuse rating, which is usually either 13a or 3a. However, 2a, 5a, and 10a fuses are available for special purposes. Cartridge fuses should be marked BS 1362. If in any doubt, ask for advice at your local Electricity Board.

BS 1362 cartridge fuses snap into the 13a plug, as it is being wired up. When a fuse "blows", it can easily be removed and replaced – *after* the plug has been removed from the socket, and *after* the electrical fault which "blew" the fuse has been rectified.

In your main fuse box, you may have any of several types of circuit overload protection fitted. Some homes are fitted with miniature circuit breakers, which snap open when overloaded. Once the fault is rectified, the circuit breaker is reset by pressing a button or switch lever.

Older systems may have wire fuses, in which a porcelain or plastic holder grips a short length of wire. The holder can be removed after switching off at the mains, and the "blown" fuse wire removed and replaced. Make absolutely certain that the proper size of fuse wire is used for the replacement: 5a for lights, 15a for heating circuits, 30a for a ring circuit. **Never** put a heavier fuse wire in to stop frequent "blowing", you risk damaging the wiring or starting a fire somewhere in the circuit.

Many modern circuits are protected with cartridge fuses (consumer unit fuses), larger versions of the fuse in a 13a plug. These, too, are simply replaced by snapping into place after switching off and rectifying the electrical fault which caused the "blown" fuse.

Checking for safety

For your own protection ensure that any new appliance has BEAB approval or complies with the appropriate British Standard, in which case the appliance will have a nameplate or ticket bearing the initials

BS followed by several numbers. Some will also have the British Standards Association "kitemark".

Items tested by the British Electrotechnical Approvals Board (BEAB), which covers most domestic appliances, whether imported or British-made, have a label attached. The approvals ensure that any appliance you buy is electrically safe to install. They cannot protect you against yourself if, for instance, you decide to dismantle the appliance to fit a longer lead, or adjust the works in any way without adequate knowledge.

Unless you know exactly what you are doing, you risk your life by making any alterations to electrical appliances. Take them to a qualified electrician for any work that needs to be done.

Here are some commonsense electrical precautions you can take yourself:

Check that the cable-clamp in each plug is tight and effective, so that strain cannot be placed on the electrical conductors or terminals.

Check that each plug is fitted with the proper-rated fuse, and that earth connections are tight.

Check that the appliance is disconnected, not just switched off, before you attempt any repairs or adjustments.

Check that electric blankets are regularly serviced, as recommended by the manufacturer.

Remember, too, that the presence of water increases the hazard of electric shock. This is why pull-cord switches and wall-mounted heaters are compulsory for bathrooms, mounted well away from puddles and splashes. Socket outlets and portable appliances must **never** be installed in bathrooms.

The same principle applies in the kitchen or elsewhere – keep portable electrical appliances away from water. This means, for instance, not using an electric mixer on the draining board, where it could fall into the sink. Even the best-designed appliance may become dangerously "live", if soaked with water.

Adaptors

A common misuse of electrical appliances in the home which can lead to fire or electric shocks is the practice of using adaptors to attach several appliances to a single socket. Used properly, an adaptor is a useful but temporary means of connecting two appliances to a socket. If you need to keep the appliances constantly plugged in, get a twin socket fitted by a professional electrician.

Using a multiple adaptor (or worse still – several adaptors) you will overload the socket mechanically if not electrically and cause overheating which could lead to a fire. You will also have an untidy "Christmas tree" of plugs which is easily pulled out from the socket when someone trips over a wire. This can damage flex or plugs and expose live connections, with a risk of serious electric shock.

Gas in the home

Properly used, gas is perfectly safe in the home. Carelessness or incorrect use, however, can be dangerous or even lethal.

Non-poisonous natural gas has now entirely replaced the old-fashioned and dangerous coal gas. But natural gas still presents the major hazards of explosion in event of a leak, and the user has a responsibility to minimise the risk.

Safety regulations

The gas safety regulations given below are legal requirements:

1. You must not use, or allow anyone else to use, any gas appliance that you know is, or might be, dangerous.

2. Only competent, properly trained people may install or service gas appliances or systems. This rules out DIY gas fitting, unless you are fully qualified.

3. You must turn off your gas at the mains if you think there is a gas leak. If gas continues to escape after turning off at the mains, you **must** (by law) tell your local gas service centre. You must not turn the gas on again until the leak has been repaired by a qualified person.

Gas leaks

If you do smell gas, there are several actions you must carry out immediately:

1. Extinguish cigarettes, and don't use matches or a naked flame.

2. Do not operate electrical switches. Turning on or *off* could cause a spark.

3. Open doors and windows wide, to allow the gas to clear.

4. Check to see if a gas tap has been left on accidentally, or a pilot light has blown out.

5. If not, there is probably a leak. Turn off the gas at the meter and telephone the gas service. There is an emergency service number under "Gas" in your local telephone directory.

6. If you cannot turn off the supply, or if the smell persists after you have turned it off, you **must** call gas service without delay.

It is dangerous to meddle with gas appliances; never attempt to repair them yourself. If ever you suspect that there is a leak, call gas service. **Never**, ever, look for a gas leak with a lighted match. This would put at risk your own life, and those of your family and neighbours.

You should know how to turn off your own main gas supply. The main tap is usually close to the gas meter. Before turning off, switch off all gas taps and pilot lights. The main tap lever should turn easily by hand. Don't use tools if it is stiff – call gas service for help. The tap is *off* when the notched line on the main spindle points across the pipe. To turn the tap *on*, the line must point along the pipe.

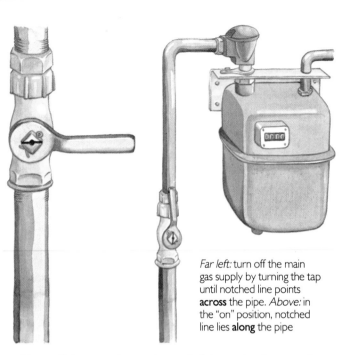

Far left: turn off the main gas supply by turning the tap until notched line points **across** the pipe. *Above:* in the "on" position, notched line lies **along** the pipe

Turn off the gas when going on holiday or leaving your home unoccupied for any length of time. Remember to relight all the pilot lights when you turn the gas back on.

Regular servicing

Make sure that you follow the instructions provided with every gas appliance, and get all appliances serviced regularly. This applies especially to central heating and to water heaters. Discolouration or staining on the walls around gas appliances may indicate that a blocked flue is causing dangerous fumes to escape. Call gas service for assistance.

Importance of ventilation

Ventilation is essential for any appliance which burns fuel — gas appliances, oil stoves, paraffin heaters and solid fuel fires must all have a proper supply of fresh air or they may produce deadly carbon monoxide fumes. It is particularly important for portable bottled gas or oil/paraffin heaters. So always ensure that, while a room does not have major draughts, some fresh air is admitted.

Many appliances must also have a chimney or flue. It is equally important that these are clear and are taking away the fumes safely to the outside atmosphere. Make sure that solid fuel fires have their chimneys swept regularly and that flued gas appliances are checked at least once a year.

Fire Prevention

Fire is an ever-present risk in the most safety-conscious home. Every room in the house contains a certain amount of flammable material, including material which may not normally burn, until preheated by other burning objects. A fire causes heat, smoke and fumes which can kill very rapidly.

Many fires occur during the night; last thing at night check that all electrical equipment not in use is switched off and unplugged. If there is an open fire, check that it is safe, and place a fireguard round it. Empty all ashtrays. Close all doors.

Though the majority of burns received in the home are minor and associated with cooking or heating appliances, each year hundreds of people – mostly children or the elderly – die from burns or scalds received in the home. Thousands more receive burns needing urgent hospital treatment, and hundreds of thousands receive more minor burns. A large proportion of those fires, burns, and scalds could have been avoided with forethought.

Potential fire hazards

Never hang kitchen curtains where they could blow over the grill or hotplate. Use blinds or non-flammable glass fibre curtaining.

Be wary of using wood panelling near the cooker and be particularly careful when using polystyrene ceiling or wall tiles in the kitchen. If you do have a fire in a chip pan, the heat will melt tiles immediately overhead, and the drips of burning plastic are extremely dangerous. Never paint polystyrene tiles with gloss paint – this can cause fire to spread rapidly.

Plastics are a fire hazard all round the house, particularly the polyether foam commonly used in upholstery. When exposed to fire, this produces dense clouds of extremely poisonous smoke which has claimed many lives. Most fires of this type are started by cigarettes and the onus is on smokers to exercise particular care. For instance, never leave a lighted cigarette in an ashtray where it could topple and start a fire. New upholstered furniture must now carry a warning label if it can be set on fire by a cigarette, match or both. After 1982 furniture must pass the cigarette test but will require labelling if it does not pass the match test.

Portable heaters, electric fires and central heating systems are all common causes of fires; all should be checked regularly to ensure that they are functioning properly. Have central heating units checked and serviced annually, and chimney or boiler flues swept regularly. Blockages can cause flames to be diverted back into the room, even though there are several built-in fail safe devices. Even more dangerous, faulty central heating units can emit poisonous or flammable gas.

Some apparently inexplicable fires start in piles of old rags or paper which have become soaked in paint, oil or wax. Under certain circumstances this material can burst into flame spontaneously, causing fires in attics, cellars, in cupboards under stairs, in sheds, or garages, where such items accumulate. *Do not wait until it happens to you, throw out such clutter now.*

Fires are often caused by drying damp clothes near to fire, or over a central heating unit, where air flow is obstructed. Remember that heavy, wet clothes may slip down and cause a fire as they dry. **Never** leave an open fire without placing a fireguard round it.

Never hang a mirror above an open fireplace where it may encourage people to lean too close.

Fire extinguishers

There are many types of fire extinguisher, and they are coded according to their usage and the chemicals they contain. If you decide to buy an extinguisher, make sure that it has a British Standards number, or Fire Extinguisher Trades Association (FETA) or Fire Offices Committee (FOC) approval.

Most of the large red fire extinguishers contain water, and are therefore dangerous if sprayed near wiring. They are seldom used in the home since there is enough water within easy access anyway.

Foam extinguishers can be used for domestic fires, although they, too, are hazardous near electricity. They are used because their smothering action is especially effective where burning liquids are involved – such as fats or oil fires.

Dry chemical extinguishers fire a spray of powder and *are probably the best general purpose extinguishers to buy for use in the home.*

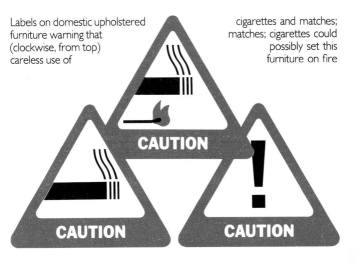

Labels on domestic upholstered furniture warning that (clockwise, from top) careless use of cigarettes and matches; matches; cigarettes could possibly set this furniture on fire

Always aim the extinguisher at the base of the fire, not at the flame or smoke. Use a side-to-side motion to blanket the burning area thoroughly. If you do have an extinguisher, keep it in the kitchen, where fires are most likely to occur. Make sure that the extinguisher is maintained regularly and recharged after use – some extinguishers are disposable and may only be used once.

It cannot be emphasised too strongly that the use of an extinguisher is no substitute for the Fire Brigade. It simply allows you to prevent a minor fire from taking hold. Having put the fire out, call the Fire Brigade by dialling 999 in all but the minor outbreaks. Fire has a habit of smouldering on long after all flames are extinguished, and it takes an expert to confirm that the risk is past.

In the car. Carry a special fire extinguisher in your car. This can be a dry powder type, or an extinguisher containing a vapourising liquid, only safe for use outdoors. Read the instructions carefully and make sure that you know how to use it – *do not* wait for an emergency to occur.

Safety in the garden

Perhaps the most dangerous single item of garden equipment is the power mower. Electric and petrol mowers pose different types of hazard, except for the rotary mower, which may have either type of power unit.

Rotary mowers have a rapidly spinning flat strip blade, under a bowl-shaped cover. The blade spins close to the ground, picking up stones or other hard objects, and firing them out in any direction, fast enough to fracture an ankle or, at the very least, to cause severe cuts on the foot and leg. It is also possible to get your toes caught under the "protective" cover causing very extensive injuries.

When using the rotary mower, take simple precautions. First pick up stones or any other obstruction from the grass. **Always** wear boots to protect feet and ankles. **Never** cut the lawn with a rotary mower while barefoot and in a swimming costume.

Most electric mowers, whether of the rotary or cylinder type, operate with a trailing power cable, usually coloured orange for visibility and with provision made for holding the cable away from the mower. But it is all too easy to run the mower over the cable, cutting it and "blowing" the fuse. The mower should already be specially insulated to avoid electrocuting the user, but **always** switch off at the mains before handling severed cable if you should run it over. **Never** attempt to mend a cut cable; take the whole mower and cable to a service agent for repair by an expert. Amateur repairs can be lethal in a cable dragging across damp grass.

Petrol mowers have very powerful motors, which are most

dangerous when the mower is out of gear, and apparently harmless. If the mower is to be left stationary for even a few minutes, stop the motor. Otherwise, the clutch may fail, allowing the machine to take off down the garden. Even more dangerous is the practice of making adjustments with the motor running but out of gear. A mechanical fault here can sever fingers.

Other potential accidents with petrol mowers are burns from the exhaust, injuries caused by the spinning flywheel, and explosive fires caused by refilling the petrol tank without stopping the motor.

The power hedge trimmer, which is usually powered by a trailing mains cable, is even more liable to accidental cuts, because it tends to get caught up and hidden in the hedge. Keep the cable slung over the shoulder opposite to the side on which you are cutting, and if the cable does get damaged, switch off the trimmer at once, put it down, and turn off at the mains. Then get it repaired professionally.

Most hedge trimmers need two-handed operation, and if you absent-mindedly release your grip with one hand, the trimmer can swivel round and gash your hand or arm. Keep the spring-loaded switch pressed down by finger pressure alone, *not locked on*, so that if you release your grip, the trimmer will just stop dead.

Use of chemicals

Garden chemicals are often poisonous; some are deadly if misused. Weedkillers, insecticides, fertilisers, etc, all need to be kept safely

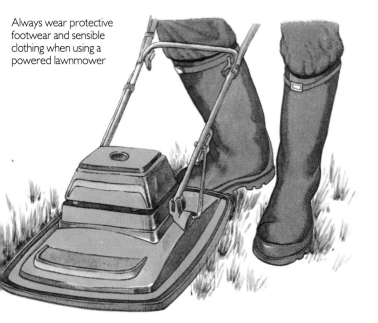

Always wear protective footwear and sensible clothing when using a powered lawnmower

locked up. When you use them, read the instructions carefully, and follow them precisely. **Never** mix garden chemicals in any household container that might be reused – keep an old bucket or tins for this purpose. To avoid accidents with unlabelled containers, dispose of any left-over chemicals immediately after you have been spraying: pour them away with plenty of water to dilute them.

When using a garden spray, always stand upwind so the mist of chemicals drifts away from you. And whenever possible choose a non-windy day for such tasks. Wash off splashes from the skin promptly, and be very wary of splashes near the eyes and mouth, which may require immediate medical attention. If you have a large garden to spray, or are spraying in an enclosed greenhouse, a simple respirator may be needed; this can be obtained from larger garden centres.

Gloves are indispensable in the garden, protecting against chemicals, cuts and thorns. Remember that deep or dirty cuts carry a risk of tetanus: seek medical advice without delay. Better still, see your doctor and get regular anti-tetanus injections *before* you have an accident – they could save your life. (A full course consists of three injections, followed by a booster injection every five years.)

D.I.Y.

The home handyman using a very wide range of tools and materials has many opportunities for accidents.

Power tools
All power tools obviously need very careful handling. Make certain they are wired up or installed properly, with the correct rating of fuse in case of overload or short circuit.

Tools such as circular saws have some form of protective shield over the blade, but no power tool can be completely safe. Many accidents are caused when the material being worked is not held securely. As it shifts, power tools can skid from the work, causing serious injury.

Protective goggles are necessary when using any form of rotary power tool: saw, grinder, drill, or wire brush. Particles of dust or wire are spun out at very high speed and can cause the loss of an eye. As with appliances for use in the garden, there is an ever-present risk of cutting through the power supply cable, so this must be kept well out of the way.

For major jobs around the home, DIY enthusiasts can hire "professional-size" power tools from the increasing number of hire shops. These are much heavier than ordinary DIY tools, and their considerable power can take the handyman by surprise, sometimes

Goggles and a respirator protect
eyes and lungs when sanding

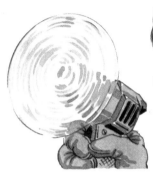
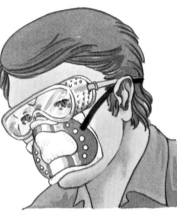

literally "running away" with him before they can be switched off.
Tools such as those used for cutting masonry produce vast amounts
of abrasive dust, and both protective goggles and a respirator **must**
be worn, otherwise both eye and lung damage could result.

Dust and fumes

Constant hazards with many forms of DIY work are dust and fumes.
Spray painting leaves paint droplets in the air, ready to be inhaled,
and also produces large amounts of explosively flammable vapour.
Good ventilation is doubly important to protect the lungs and reduce
fire risks. If there is the slightest doubt about the ventilation, use a
respirator mask.

Sanding dust is a lung and eye irritant too, and if inhaled in large
amounts can cause lung disease. Yet another lung hazard is the
asbestos composition sheet sometimes used for roofing. Intact, it is
quite safe but, when sawn or sanded, asbestos particles may be
inhaled with extremely dangerous results. Glass fibre insulation, too,
needs great care in handling.

When sanding, sawing, or spraying indoors, try to use some form
of dust extraction. An electric fan can be used to blow dust and
fumes out of a window, or if you have a powerful vacuum cleaner
this can be left running nearby to remove dust as it is produced.

Cutting and boring tools

Cuts and abrasions are often caused by tools of this type when the
work piece shifts unexpectedly. Make sure that the work is securely
fixed by clamps or a vice when drilling, planing, sawing and,
particularly, when using a chisel. Very bad injuries can be caused by a
slipping chisel, which usually has all your weight behind it. And
remember, **always** cut away from you when using a chisel or any
other sharp-edged tool.

Ladders

Ladders are used by most handymen, and must be kept in good repair. Extension ladders in particular need good maintenance. Make sure they are firmly placed on a level surface, and if the base has an anti-slip device, be sure it is used properly.

Car maintenance

Here, DIY introduces some special problems. It is not good practice to work around the engine while it is running, but this is sometimes unavoidable. If you have to make adjustments or repairs, try to wear gloves, and make sure you have no loose clothing such as a tie which could catch on the fan belt and pull you into contact with the engine.

Burns are common when working on cars. Scalds result from contact with near-boiling water in the radiator, but burns from the exhaust or manifold can be much worse, due to the higher temperatures involved.

Although only low voltages are present in a car electrical system, extremely high currents are produced in short circuits, such as can be made inadvertently when using a spanner or screwdriver while the ignition is switched on. The current can melt a screwdriver blade, and an incautious hand can be showered with sparks of red-hot metal. You could receive a painful electric shock if you are working with the high-tension part of the ignition system.

Removing wheels puts a very heavy strain on an ordinary car jack. Always use axle stand ramps, or a proper garage jack if the car is to be supported for any length of time, especially if it is necessary to work under the car – **never** balance the car on bricks, which crumble under the weight.

Safety for children

Children are the most vulnerable members of the family. When very young, they are helpless to protect themselves against everyday hazards, and are susceptible to accidents that seldom affect adults, such as suffocation by their bedding.

The baby lying in a cot may be unable to turn himself over if his breathing becomes restricted. So give him either no pillow at all, or a firm, thin pillow, to prevent smothering when he turns face-down. **Do not** use polythene sheeting to protect the cot mattress – it is totally airtight and can block a child's breathing.

Similarly, the baby's air passages are easily blocked by small objects, or by small amounts of vomited food. **Do not** give a baby any object small enough to put in his mouth, and **do not** leave him unattended with a bottle propped up so that he can feed himself.

As he gets older and more mobile, the enquiring mind of the child leads to new problems, and falls, scalds, cuts, burns and poisoning become serious hazards.

Preventing falls

As soon as the baby begins to crawl, or even to roll about on his own, falls become a special hazard. A stair gate is essential when baby first begins to explore. But sooner or later it may be left open accidentally, and the baby will inevitably explore the stairs. To avoid the risk of falls, as soon as baby can crawl confidently, teach him how to climb the stairs, and how to come down backwards.

Nappy changing is a frequent cause of falls, when a baby wriggles unexpectedly off the knees, or rolls off a table. It is safer to put the baby in the middle of a bed for changing.

Other more dangerous falls are associated with prams, pushchairs, carrycots, and high chairs, which the baby may manage to overbalance with himself in it. The weight of a falling pram or pushchair is considerable, but neither should be capable of tipping, unless overloaded with a heavy shopping bag, or parked carelessly.

Use restraint straps in prams, pushchairs and high chairs to prevent head-first falls if the baby tries to climb out.

Preventing burns and scalds

When the child can crawl or walk, part of his exploration of the environment is to reach out and touch any familiar or unfamiliar object. This is the chief cause of burns and scalds in early childhood.

Use a fixed fireguard around any type of fire, and make sure it is "safety approved", with only small spaces between the protective grille. Still keep a close watch on baby to make sure he doesn't try to push pencils or any other thin objects through the holes in the grille.

For the child, there is a high risk of burns and scalds in the kitchen. To prevent them is relatively easy, but this does involve you in constant vigilance. A child will unhesitatingly grasp dangerous objects which an adult would never think of touching. Cups of hot drinks, teapots, and toasters left within reach of a child sat at the kitchen table, can produce severe scalds or burns. Do not use a tablecloth, as by pulling on the cloth the child can tip hot food or tea over himself.

Splashes of boiling water and spits of fat are both likely to fall on a small child standing unnoticed close to the cooker, so keep children well away when cooking is in progress.

Scalds can happen when baby's bathwater is not checked for the correct temperature. **Never** add more hot water while baby is in the bath. Check hot-water bottles carefully for leaks, and wrap them in a thick protective cover. **Never** leave the hot-water bottle in the cot or bed with the baby.

A baby's questing small fingers make him very liable to electric shocks. Blank off unused wall sockets with dummy plugs, or seal them with adhesive tape. You can buy special 13a plugs which have the metal pins partly sheathed with insulation, so that even if they are slightly pulled out from the socket, it is impossible to touch "live" metal.

Pay special attention to the state of appliance leads where they leave the plug. Make certain that the plug grips the outer insulation firmly, and is not just attached by the thin vulnerable inner wires.

If you use an electric cot blanket, switch off and unplug it **before** putting the baby to bed. Even an isolated case of bedwetting could cause electrocution.

Poisonous substances

Anything which comes to hand finishes up in the mouth of an exploring child. Keep *everything* which a child might eat or drink – even shoe polish and soap – locked away or well out of reach. Obvious poisons like bleach, oven cleaner, and medicines must be locked securely away.

Nowadays toys are made to rigorous safety standards, but a few dangerous examples still slip through – usually imported. Check for security of toys' eyes and any other easily swallowed small parts, and make sure painted toys have a "non-toxic" label to avoid poisoning.

Outdoor hazards

Poisonous plants are a subject in themselves, and a large number of common garden plants and shrubs are extremely dangerous if eaten. Be especially cautious with the seed pods of laburnum, which look like miniature pea pods, and fascinate children, with possibly fatal results. And **always** lock the garden shed; it is full of potential hazards.

If you have a swing in the garden, make sure that it has a secure

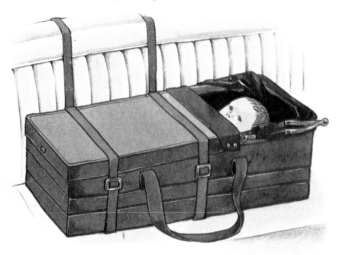

seat frame in which the child can sit without risk of falling. Never let your child near the old-fashioned swing with a heavy plank seat, which can cause terrible injuries if it swings back against the child.

Water is a magnet for any curious child. Uncovered water butts, and unfenced streams, and ponds are all hazards – a small child can drown quickly in only a couple of inches of water.

Family pets

Children should be taught how to handle pets to avoid bites and scratches. Also try to prevent pets from licking your child's face, as such close contact can spread worms or other diseases.

Cover the pram with a net if you have a cat or there are cats in the neighbourhood – this is necessary even indoors with a cot or carrycot. Young babies are easily suffocated by a cat seeking a warm and comfortable place to sleep.

Car safety

It is now illegal to allow a child to sit on the lap of a front seat passenger – quite rightly, as in a collision the child goes through the windscreen or is crushed against the instrument panel.

Fit a special child's safety harness in the back of the car, and always use it. Babies can be safely tucked in a carrycot securely strapped into the back of the car.

Children old enough to sit comfortably upright receive a good deal of protection even from adult-sized seat belts, and it is safer to allow such a child to sit strapped in, on the front passenger seat, rather than in the back, with no seat belt.

Always set child-proof car locks, if these are fitted, and if the child is left alone in the car for even a few minutes make sure that ignition keys have been removed and the handbrake is firmly on.

Always use the appropriate safety harness when travelling with children

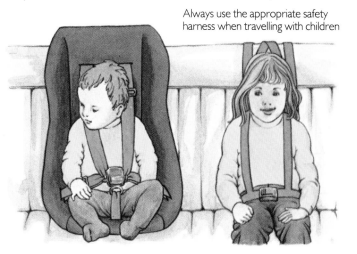

Safety for the elderly and infirm

All types of accidents become more common for the elderly, and among the most frequent, and certainly the most dangerous, is a fall.

Falls, like other accidents for the elderly, result from the normal effects of ageing. As senses become less effective, the elderly may no longer have fast enough reflexes to prevent an accident. The sense of balance is one of the worst affected, sometimes causing an elderly person to fall without any apparent reason. Falls are dangerous as with increasing age the bones become brittle, and even a heavy bone like the femur in the thigh may break after a minor fall.

Preventing falls

All the usual commonsense precautions against slipping and tripping over must be taken, to help protect the elderly. But because the risks are so much higher, some additional measures can be useful.

1. Fit handrails on *both* sides of the staircase.
2. Fit extra-strong light bulbs in hallways, passages, and on staircases.
3. Use a special non-slip mat in the bath and on the bathroom floor. Falls in the bathroom are particularly dangerous as the head is likely to strike the bath, sink, or toilet. Here, too, special handrails are useful, above the bath and alongside the toilet.
4. If an elderly or infirm person finds walking difficult, or their balance is badly impaired, persuade them to contact the Social Services or WRVS to borrow a walking frame.

Keeping warm

Heating is critically important for the elderly, as the state of "hypothermia", or reduced body heat, can be very dangerous. An old person may not even realise that their home is too cold, and can gradually sink into a sleepy and confused state which may be fatal if they are not found in time.

If you suspect that an old person you know is not keeping warm enough, make some tactful enquiries. If you find there is a problem – perhaps they may not be able to afford to heat their home – contact the Social Services yourself and ask them to call. At-risk elderly people may be eligible for a special heating allowance.

Medicines

Many old people need to take several different kinds of medicine, and it is a matter of concern to doctors that they often become confused about which tablet to take, at particular times of day. It may be helpful to measure out all their day's tablets into separate containers, clearly marked "morning", "lunchtime", "evening", and "bedtime". This ensures that all the tablets are taken at the proper time, and reduces the chance of absent-mindedly taking too many.

There are many well-designed
aids to ensure bathroom safety

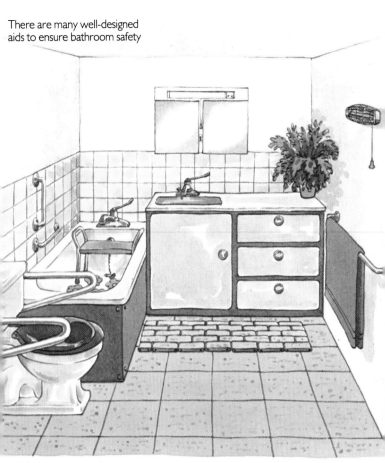

Left: well-lit staircase and hallway

Walking-frame assists mobility

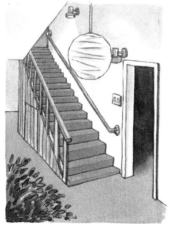

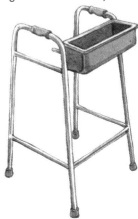

2: Dealing with an Emergency

ACTION PRIORITIES

In any emergency it is essential that you remain calm. After an accident, you must rapidly assess the degree of injury, and decide on the measures which need to be taken. If you behave in a calm, confident manner you will reassure the casualty and win the co-operation of bystanders.

Examination check-list

Quickly and methodically examine the casualty to assess the extent of his injuries. This should be done as far as possible with the casualty in the position in which he was found. In any case, **do not** turn an unconscious casualty on to his back.

1. Check – is the casualty breathing? If *not*, turn to page 42 immediately.
2. Check – is he bleeding? Feel carefully over and under for dampness.
3. Then, starting at the head, look for any wounds. Speak to casualty and assess level of consciousness. Try to reassure him – even if he is unconscious, he may be able to hear you.
4. Check the pupils. Are they "pinpoint" or unequal?
5. Check for bleeding from ears, nose or mouth.
6. Check for fluid, froth, burns and stains to the mouth. Remove any potential obstruction from airways e.g. dentures.
7. Check for any odour on breath.
8. Examine the rest of body: neck, spine, trunk, arms and legs, feeling with the flat of your hand.
9. An unconscious casualty should be searched for medical cards e.g. Diabetic, Steroid or Anti-coagulent card.
10. Take the pulse, noting rate, rhythm, strength.

If the injury is minor, you may reasonably decide to treat it yourself. If not, first aid must be given *as an interim measure only*, until proper medical treatment can be provided.

Having assessed the immediate needs in dealing with the accident, enlist the aid of anyone who is nearby, provided they appear able to cope calmly with whatever needs to be done.

If the injury is not serious, get someone to organise car transport to hospital, and remember that a roomy car is preferable, so that the casualty can be comfortable. Travel with him in case emergency treatment proves necessary.

If the accident is more serious, telephone the emergency services, by dialling 999, and when the operator replies, ask for "ambulance". Always give the number of the telephone from which you are calling, and the address or exact location of the place where the casualty is being given first aid. If this is not possible, mention any prominent landmark e.g. church, cinema, public house, garage, bridge, etcetera. Give brief details of the type of accident and the condition of the casualty or casualties – see examination check-list opposite.

If the casualty has been badly injured and you have to undertake immediate first aid, send a helper to make the 999 call.

Never give a badly injured person food or drink. He may become unconscious or, if he has to be operated on, need a general anaesthetic. In either event, on a full stomach he could vomit or choke.

The only exceptions are:

1. Anyone who has been badly burnt may have small sips of water.

2. Anyone who has swallowed corrosive poison should be given tepid water (milk if available) in small sips.

In either case **do not** attempt to give liquids if the casualty is unconscious.

Always protect the casualty from cold and reassure him that the situation is under control. Do not keep asking him how he feels as this would add to the stress he is already undergoing. If he enquires about others possibly injured in the same accident, reassure him that they are being cared for.

Fire

Your immediate priorities in the event of fire are to get all the occupants out of the building, close all doors and windows as you leave to prevent the fire from spreading, and call the Fire Brigade by dialling 999. Then stay well clear.

Small fires can be extinguished with water (except where live electrical equipment is the cause), by smothering them with a rug, or use of a fire extinguisher. Be very careful if there is a lot of smoke, as you may be overcome by fumes.

Do not continue to fight a fire if:

1. The fire spreads despite your efforts.

2. There is a risk that your escape route may be cut off by fire or smoke.

If you are trapped

If you are unlucky enough to be trapped in the house, don't be in a hurry to open the door to escape. First check whether it feels warm, or smoke is coming round the edges. In either event **do not** open the door under any circumstances.

Try to block off the smoke with carpet, curtains, or clothing. Stay near the window until help arrives and **do not** jump unless instructed to do so. If the smoke gets bad, lie on the floor where the air is clearer (with a damp cloth over your face, if possible).

If a casualty's clothes are burning, lay him down and smother the flames with coats, rugs or blankets. **Do not** roll him round and round as this would expose even more of his body to the flames.

Treat BURNS as described on page 66; SHOCK as on page 50.

Fires in cooking pans can be extinguished by covering them with a lid or a damp cloth.

Never use water.

Never try to pick up a burning pan. First extinguish the fire, then get rid of the smoking pan when it has cooled.

Fires in ovens are best handled by closing the oven door.

In either emergency, turn off all the cooker taps.

Electrical fires need special treatment, as heat generated by the electricity keeps the fire burning. Switch off at the main, then unplug the burning appliance before attempting to extinguish the fire. Once you've switched off at the main water can be used safely.

Always call the Fire Brigade to check after extinguishing electrical fires in wall sockets, as insulation may still be smouldering.

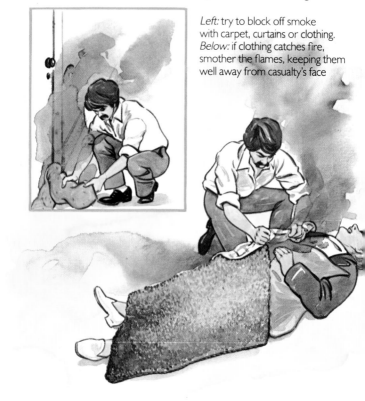

Left: try to block off smoke with carpet, curtains or clothing.
Below: if clothing catches fire, smother the flames, keeping them well away from casualty's face

Carbon monoxide poisoning

Now that coal gas has been fully replaced by natural gas, a major cause of carbon monoxide poisoning has been removed. But several other sources still remain.

Car exhaust fumes are perhaps the best known, but defective household heating appliances can also be a hazard.

Carbon monoxide is odourless and colourless. It does not occur naturally, only being produced when any fuel is incorrectly burned. Petrol, oil, paraffin, gas, solid fuel, even wood – all can produce dangerous fumes containing carbon monoxide.

The symptoms of carbon monoxide poisoning are easily mistaken for other ailments. Unexplained headaches, nausea and lassitude are the first signs. A victim in more serious cases will appear confused and sleepy, and perhaps become unconscious.

To give effective help, speed is vital:

1. Before attempting to reach the casualty, take several deep breaths of fresh air yourself – and hold your breath while in the gas-filled room or car. **Otherwise you put your own life at risk.** If there is more than one casualty, repeat this action before each return to the gas-filled area.

2. Get the casualty into the fresh air.

3. Turn off any appliances that are burning in the room. If a car exhaust has caused the accident, switch off the engine.

4. Open all windows and doors wide to allow toxic fumes to disperse quickly.

5. Give emergency treatment as required. See UNCONSCIOUS-NESS, page 41 and ARTIFICIAL RESPIRATION, page 44.

6. Dial 999 for an ambulance and call Gas Service if there has been a leakage from domestic gas supplies – the telephone number is prominently displayed under GAS in all local telephone directories.

7. Prevent bystanders from smoking.

Asphyxiation

A difficult word for a simple, but deadly, situation. It means that a person is not getting sufficient air to breathe and therefore cannot live. A variety of causes can deprive the normal atmosphere of fresh air, and this is more likely in confined places such as sewers and wells. Casualties, once rescued, should be treated in exactly the same way as for carbon monoxide poisoning.

It is vitally important that, if you attempt to rescue a person trapped in a septic tank, well or sewer, you must have a safety rope attached to you and you must have several helpers. If at all possible, wait for the arrival of those who are specially trained and equipped for the task. Tragically, amateur rescuers all too often die in their well-meaning attempts.

Electric shock

Electricity can cause serious injuries, from burns to upsetting the pulse rate and causing death. Shock can also have serious delayed effects on the casualty. It is essential for the rescuer to exercise great care, and ensure that he does not touch a casualty still in contact with electrical wires or terminals.

Accidents caused by high tension cables or railway conductor rails: if the casualty is thrown clear by the shock, treatment for severe BURNS (page 66), and ARTIFICIAL RESPIRATION (page 44) can be given without delay.

If they remain in contact with the high tension current **under no circumstances even approach them**. Keep at least 18.3 m (20 yards) away to be safe. *Do not* attempt to move the casualty clear with a piece of wood or any other object, as the current can bridge a considerable gap and your own life will be at risk.

Dial 999 and ask for Ambulance Service. Explain the full situation and all the necessary services will be despatched automatically. Return to the site of the accident and stay there to point out the spot, **but do nothing further**.

Accidents caused by domestic electrical supply: these, too, can be very dangerous to the rescuer if insufficient care is taken when handling the casualty.

Your first objective is to separate the casualty from the current.
1. Break the electrical contact by switching off or unplugging the current, either at the socket or, if this cannot be safely reached, by turning off at the mains. **Do not** touch the casualty or his clothes until this has been done.
2. If you cannot disconnect the supply, make sure that you are standing on a dry floor, to prevent any possibility of current being earthed through your body. If the floor is damp, stand on a piece of dry wood or cardboard.
3. Even then, do not touch the casualty with bare hands; use an insulated object to move him away. Use a piece of wood such as a walking stick, rolled newspapers or a bundle of clothing. Sometimes, a clothesline can be looped around the casualty, so that he can be dragged clear.

The casualty will probably need ARTIFICIAL RESPIRATION (page 44).

The current has a serious effect on the heart, and HEART MASSAGE may also be needed (page 46).

There will almost certainly be electrical BURNS. These may look insignificant but they are often very deep and may have serious after effects (page 66).

Sometimes, there are BROKEN BONES (page 61) caused by sudden muscle contraction due to the electric shock.

Dial 999 for an ambulance without delay. After *any* electric shock, expert medical treatment is essential.

Car accidents

If you are in your own car when you witness, or come upon, an accident of this nature, first park your own car safely, with hazard lights on, if you have them.

Remember that there is still a hazard due to other traffic. **Do not** rush across the road to the crashed car, injured cyclist or pedestrian. Make sure that it is safe to approach, and if you have someone with you get him to direct traffic around the scene of the accident. If hazard triangles are available, place them in the roadway.

Keep bystanders well back, unless there are people among them who can help. In any car crash, prevent helpers and bystanders from smoking, to minimise fire hazard.

Turn off the ignition.

If there are several casualties, check rapidly to see who requires first aid most urgently. **Do not** try to get casualties out of a crashed car until you have determined the extent of their injuries, unless there is an obvious fire hazard. You could do more harm than good. *If they are unconscious or have spinal injuries, leave them in the car until medical help arrives*, but make sure they can breathe by supporting the head.

If there is not a telephone box nearby, stop a passing motorist – better still, stop two going in opposite directions – and ask both to telephone for the emergency services. Make sure that they each have all the relevant information:
1. The location of the accident.
2. Number injured and extent of injuries.
3. Whether anyone is trapped.

Never attempt to move a car in order to lift a casualty clear, however necessary this may be, without having adequate help to move it safely.

If a motorcyclist is the casualty, **do not** remove the crash-helmet unless his airways are blocked.

Keep the casualty warm and do not move him more than necessary. Usually a casualty will instinctively adopt the position most natural to his comfort.

Treat injuries as described in the appropriate section of this book, bearing in mind that, even if conscious, the casualty may be in shock and oblivious to pain from a wound not immediately obvious. **Proceed with great care**.

Drowning

In drowning, the lungs and air passages become blocked or partly filled with water, or frothy mucus. First aid is intended to supply air to the lungs, restore breathing and make sure that the heart is beating. **Do not** try to drain water from the lungs; this will be expelled when the casualty starts to cough, as breathing is restored. Begin MOUTH TO MOUTH RESUSCITATION (page 44) in the water if possible. Only the casualty's head need be above water. Continue artificial respiration while the casualty is being pulled ashore. Otherwise, carry out artificial respiration on the beach, or in a boat. **Do not** wait until the casualty can be carried indoors or made more comfortable.

Continue with mouth-to-mouth resuscitation until medical help arrives. **Do not** give up, even after an hour. When the casualty starts to breathe, be prepared to continue mouth-to-mouth resuscitation until normal strong breathing is restored. Then turn the casualty into the RECOVERY POSITION (page 41). Be ready to recommence artificial respiration if breathing weakens.

The casualty must be removed to hospital urgently; even after apparent recovery there may be serious lung inflammation.

While waiting for an ambulance to arrive make sure that the casualty is kept warm, as hypothermia (page 67) is a possible hazard after even a short immersion in cold water.

See also BREATHING PROBLEMS, page 42. CHOKING, page 68.

Do not delay. Begin resuscitation in the water and continue as casualty is pulled ashore

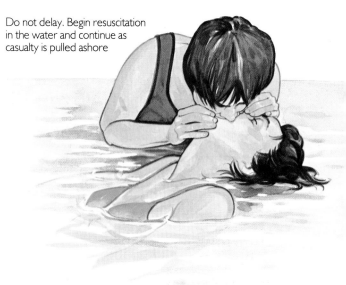

Childbirth in an emergency

When birth contractions begin, there is usually adequate time to get the expectant mother to hospital, or for the doctor or midwife to attend.

Occasionally, however, the birth comes on very quickly, or other circumstances prevent normal medical help from being available. The techniques for helping deliver the baby described below are intended **only for such emergencies**, and are no substitute for professional medical care.

If an emergency delivery does seem imminent, *do not panic*. The baby would probably be born easily without any help. But as you are there, you can make things easier by ensuring cleanliness, and reassuring the mother.

First, send for medical help: an ambulance if the mother is booked in for a hospital delivery; the doctor, or the midwife.

An early symptom of imminent delivery is a low, nagging backache. This is normally followed by a "show", or discharge of blood-stained mucus, indicating that the birth canal is beginning to widen ready for the passage of the baby.

Regular wavelike contractions in the lower abdomen are unmistakable signs that the birth process is under way, as is the "breaking of the waters" when the protective membranes around the baby rupture, releasing a pint or more of clear fluid.

Get the mother to bed, or lying comfortably on a clean level surface. Make sure you have ready all the items you will need. There should be plenty of time, as birth is normally an extended process.

Items required

1. A clean blanket, towel, or shawl in which to wrap the baby.

2. A cot. If you have to improvise, a drawer or even a box lined with a blanket will suffice.

3. Sharp scissors which have been boiled for 10 minutes to sterilise them, for cutting the cord.

4. Three pieces of string, each about 23 cm (9 inches) long, for tying the cord. Sterilise them by boiling for 10 minutes.

5. Adequate hot water, 2 basins or bowls, clean swabs, and plastic or strong paper bags in which to place soiled swabs.

Cover the bed with a waterproof sheet or, if this is not available, with several layers of newspaper. Cover with a clean sheet or large towels.

Have an additional clean sheet and towels available to cover the top part of the mother's body during the delivery.

Scrupulous cleanliness is essential.

Wash your hands thoroughly: scrub them, preferably under running water if this is possible, and clean well under the nails. Let them dry naturally – *do not* use a towel. If your hands become soiled, wash them again.

If the mother has received detailed instructions about the birth from her antenatal clinic, let her follow them, and restrict your actions to helping at her request.

Birth takes place in three distinct stages

First stage: this normally lasts for a few hours, but can be much shorter, especially in women who have already borne a child. During this stage, the womb or uterus contracts once every 10 to 20 minutes, the contractions increasing in regularity until they occur every few minutes.

This happens automatically, and the mother should try to remain relaxed. She should *not* bear down at this point.

Early on, between contractions, the mother should empty her bladder and try to move her bowels.

Second stage: actual birth often commences with a rush of fluid, the "breaking of the waters". The mother now has a very strong urge to push or bear down. She will find it helpful to lie on her back, with her legs drawn up, and grip behind her knees with her hands. As each contraction begins, she should breathe deeply in and out, then take another deep breath and hold it. This helps the womb to contract strongly. Between contractions she should lie back and try to rest.

Soon a bulge will appear, as the baby's head nears the end of the birth canal. *Birth is now beginning.*

Unless the mother has been instructed otherwise by the doctor or clinic, turn her onto her left side, with her knees drawn up, and her buttocks near the edge of the bed. Give her a pillow to support her head, and keep her body warm by covering the top half with towels wrapped inside a folded clean sheet. It is possible that the strong contractions will cause an involuntary bowel movement. If so, clean carefully, wiping away from front to back to avoid soiling the birth canal.

The mother should now *stop* bearing down, and breathe in short, shallow pants, with her mouth open, to slow the birth process slightly.

The baby's head should begin to emerge slowly. Sometimes an arm or leg may appear first. Support the head gently in the palm of the hand as it emerges. **Do not** pull.

Take no other action except when:

1. There is a membrane over the baby's face (the "caul"). This must be torn away gently, to allow the baby to breathe.

2. The thick "cord" is looped round the baby's neck. Try to manoeuvre it over the head or shoulder to prevent the baby's blood supply from being affected. Under **no** circumstances pull on the cord.

The next few contractions deliver the head and shoulders. Hold the baby *gently but firmly* beneath the armpits – he may emerge quite suddenly, and will be very slippery. Lift the baby clear, and lie him down near the mother's abdomen. *Take great care not to stretch or pull the cord.*

Wrap a clean cloth round the baby's ankles, and *grip them firmly*, with a finger locked between the ankles. Pick him up, so that he is suspended head downwards. Using the other hand, gently wipe away blood and mucus from around his mouth and nose; open his mouth to let fluid drain out.

He should start to cry within a few moments. If he shows no sign of crying or breathing within two minutes, start mouth-to-mouth and nose respiration (page 45). Blow very gently, to avoid damage. **Do not** slap the baby to start him breathing.

In a breech delivery, where the baby emerges bottom-first, the birth should still proceed normally. Only after the shoulders and arms have emerged and if the baby's head remains inside the mother for three more minutes should his body be pulled *very gently and steadily* to help delivery.

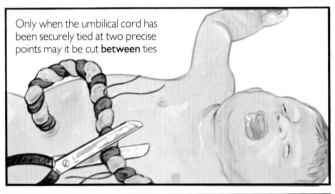

Only when the umbilical cord has been securely tied at two precise points may it be cut **between** ties

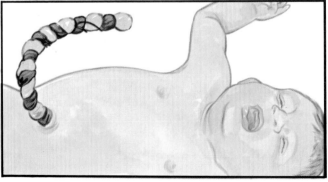

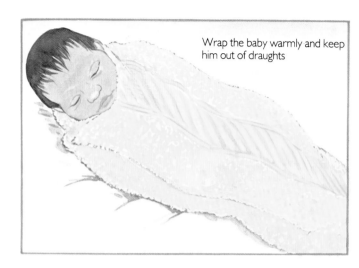

Wrap the baby warmly and keep him out of draughts

Do not touch or interfere with the cord.

Lay the mother comfortably on her back, and give her the warmly wrapped baby to hold while you prepare for the third stage.

Third stage: usually between 5 and 10 minutes after delivery, the afterbirth (tissue mass by which the foetus was nourished within the womb) will be expelled by further contractions, and by the mother bearing down. It usually emerges without difficulty. If there is much bleeding, massage the mother's abdomen gently, to stimulate contraction of the womb. This can be felt just below the navel.

The cord must be tied off 10 minutes after the baby is born, whether or not the afterbirth has emerged.

Tie two pieces of sterilised string **very securely** around the cord, one at about 15 cm (6 inches), and the second 20 cm (8 inches) from the baby's navel.

Using the sterilised scissors, cut the cord **between** the two knots. Put a sterile, dry dressing over the baby's end of the cord. *Do not* use powder or disinfectant of any kind. After 10 minutes check to make sure that bleeding has stopped, then securely tie the third piece of sterilised string around the cord 10 cm (4 inches) from the baby's navel.

Wrap the baby in a clean towel, shawl or blanket, and keep him out of draughts.

Retain the afterbirth in a covered basin for the doctor to examine later.

Now wash the mother and help her to put on a fresh nightdress. Give her an absorbent sanitary towel – not internal protection. Make her comfortable, give her a hot drink, and allow her to rest.

Then, even if the birth has been without problem, contact the doctor without further delay.

TREATMENT PRIORITIES

Unconsciousness

Many accidents can lead to unconsciousness, and special first aid procedures for many of these are described in this book, but your first priority must be to preserve life by ensuring that the casualty is breathing properly.

Use your fingers to remove any obstructions from the mouth: dentures, food, vomit, blood, or broken teeth. Use a handkerchief to remove remaining blood or vomit.

Loosen clothing at neck, chest and waist. Remove glasses, if worn.

Turn the casualty into the RECOVERY POSITION, described below, unless he is so badly injured that it would be dangerous to move him, in which case try to turn his head to one side. First, kneel beside him and place both his arms close to his body. Then cross his far arm and leg over his body and pull the far hip over so that he is lying on his side – protecting his head with your free hand as you do so. If help is available, and the casualty heavy, ask the helper to cradle the casualty's head as you turn him.

Now place the casualty's top arm and leg at right angles and tilt his head slightly back with his chin jutting out to keep his tongue clear of the back of his throat.

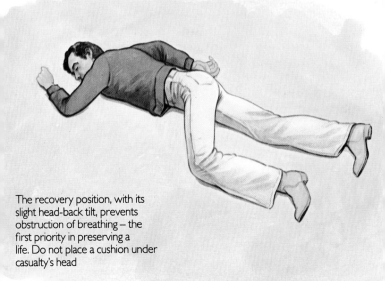

The recovery position, with its slight head-back tilt, prevents obstruction of breathing – the first priority in preserving a life. Do not place a cushion under casualty's head

Loosen any restrictive clothing but keep the casualty warm.

If you have been able to place the casualty on a bed, raise the bottom of the bed by about 30 cm (1 ft). The resulting slight head-down position helps to drain fluids out of the air passages.

Keep a close watch on the casualty while waiting for medical aid. He may vomit, or his breathing may deteriorate to the point where he needs ARTIFICIAL RESPIRATION (page 44).

All unconscious casualties must be seen by a doctor, even if they appear to recover spontaneously. Do not allow them to drink or eat until they have been seen by a doctor.

Breathing problems

Failure of breathing is a serious emergency and demands immediate and correct first aid measures to preserve life. Call 999 for Ambulance Service, as continuous lack of oxygen is rapidly fatal and even short periods of suffocation can cause brain damage.

Typical accidents which can cause stoppage of breathing are: head injuries, unconsciousness, gassing, electric shock, drowning, choking and poisoning.

Breathing may stop because of a blockage in the air passages, or because due to some malfunction, the brain is no longer issuing the correct "breathing" instructions to the chest and trunk muscles.

If a casualty appears not to be breathing, check **quickly** before commencing first aid. Listen at the casualty's lips and nose, and try to feel a current of air. Watch to see if the chest rises and falls, or feel the stomach just below the ribs, to see if it rises and falls due to breathing.

Check for signs of breathing by listening at casualty's lips and nose and watching to see if chest rises and falls

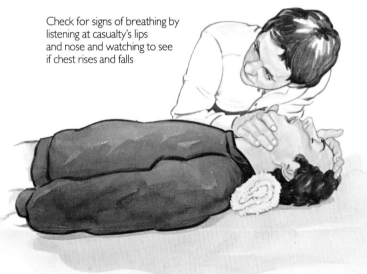

If the casualty is not breathing, you have less than five minutes in which to start the breathing again. Otherwise, permanent brain damage or death follows quickly.

Obstructions to breathing: air passages can become blocked naturally if a person is deeply unconscious, as the tongue drops back into the throat. This usually happens if the casualty is lying on his back.

The blockage may be caused by: vomit, blood, loose dentures, or large pieces of food. Quickly remove any obvious obstructions from the casualty's mouth. Reach well into the back of the throat with your fingers to ensure that nothing is still wedged there. At this point, many casualties begin to breathe again without further help.

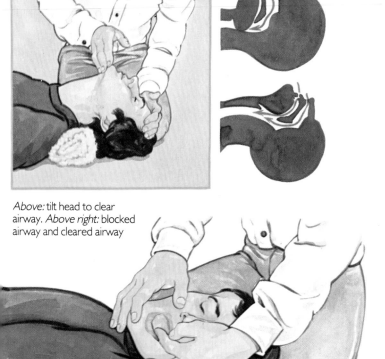

Above: tilt head to clear airway. *Above right:* blocked airway and cleared airway

Clearing obstructions from the mouth of an unconscious casualty

If breathing has not started, roll the casualty onto his back and tilt his head well back by lifting his chin – holding him firmly below the chin and by the top of the head. This will lift the tongue away from the back of his throat leaving a clear airway.

Loosen clothing at the neck, chest and waist.

Check **quickly** to see if breathing has started. If not, begin artificial respiration **immediately**.

Artificial respiration

In adults, use the mouth-to-mouth technique ("kiss of life"); for children, use mouth-to-mouth and nose.

Mouth-to-mouth: hold the casualty's head fully extended, as described above, pinch the casualty's nostrils shut between your finger and thumb, take a deep breath, then seal your lips firmly around his mouth. Blow out steadily into the casualty's mouth, until the chest rises as air enters the lungs.

Remove your mouth, and watch the chest fall again.

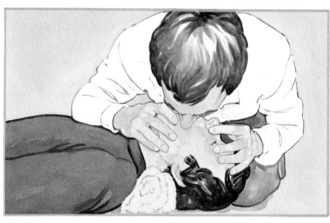

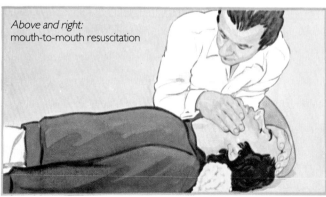

Above and right:
mouth-to-mouth resuscitation

Continue the cycle of blowing into his mouth and watching his chest rise and fall, at a comfortable natural rate of breathing.

If the chest does not rise and fall, or there is resistance to breathing into the casualty's mouth, there is probably still an obstruction in the throat. Check again.

Turn the casualty onto his side, still with his head held well back, and thump him sharply on the back, between his shoulder blades. Remove dislodged material from the mouth and resume artificial respiration.

Mouth-to-mouth and nose: in babies and young children, place your lips over both mouth and nose together.

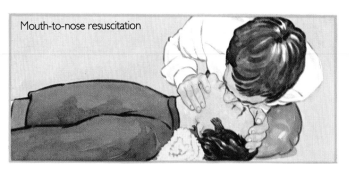

Mouth-to-nose resuscitation

Blow gently into the lungs and watch for the chest to rise. Otherwise, proceed exactly as for adults.

Continue artificial respiration until the casualty is breathing normally, then place him in the RECOVERY POSITION (page 41), and send for an ambulance.

It is important to lay the casualty on his side, exactly as in the illustration, with his head turned to one side to prevent possible inhalation of vomit during recovery.

Keep a watch on the casualty until help arrives, to make sure that breathing continues unaided. If breathing difficulties recur, resume the artificial respiration immediately.

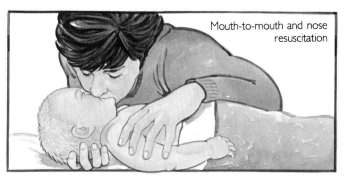

Mouth-to-mouth and nose resuscitation

Heart Failure

What to do if the heart stops. If the heart stops beating, or beats with a weak, quivery action, there is immediate risk to life.

Because he is not breathing, the casualty will already be a bluish-grey colour. After only a few breaths of artificial respiration, this colour should improve. But if the casualty remains bluish-grey, the heart may no longer be functioning properly. A further sign is that the pupils of the eyes become dilated and do not contract when the eyelids are held open.

Another indication of heart failure is that the pulse in the side of the neck cannot be felt, although this may not be apparent to an inexperienced first-aider if the heart is beating only weakly.

Lay the casualty flat on his back, and thump the chest hard with the side of the hand, towards lower end of the breastbone, and slightly to the left of his chest. The heart may start to beat again without further treatment. If not, repeat once or twice.

In babies, use two fingers to give a sharp tap on the chest; this should restart the heart.

In either case, adult or baby, if this simple first aid measure does not work, external heart massage (also called heart compression) will be needed. This is more difficult, and if it were carried out while the heart was still beating, *serious damage could be caused. Check carefully* the three important signs that the heart is not working:
1. Blue-grey skin colour.
2. Dilated pupils (i.e. over-sized pupils).
3. Lack of pulse beat.

Carry out heart massage (heart compression) as follows:
Kneel to one side of the casualty, locate the lower end of the breastbone. Place the heel of one hand on the chest near the centre of the breastbone, with the fingers and palm lifted clear of the chest. Place your other hand over this hand, again resting on the heel of the hand.

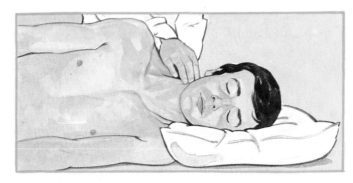

Hold your arms stiff, then rock your body forward to press down on the casualty's breastbone, which should press in (in an adult) by about 3.5 to 5 cm (1½ to 2 inches).

Rock your body back to let the breastbone rise, then repeat the whole manoeuvre, in a smooth rhythm.

In adults, press at a rate of about 60 times each minute.

In children, *press more gently,* with one hand only – but faster, about 80 to 90 times each minute.

In babies, use only two fingers for compression, and press higher, towards the middle of the breastbone. *Press very lightly* and quickly, at 100 times each minute.

In all cases, avoid violent movement which could cause internal injury.

Restarting of the heart is shown by a rapid recovery of more normal colour, normal responses of the pupils, and return of the pulse in the side of the neck.

Ideally, you should have someone to continue with artificial respiration while you carry out heart massage at the rate of six compressions to each rapid breath of artificial respiration. If you have to do it single-handed, give 15 heart compressions followed by two *rapid* breaths of artificial respiration.

Both artificial respiration and/or heart compression need to be continued until either a doctor or ambulance crew can take over, or the casualty is obviously recovering.

When the heart is beating satisfactorily, and breathing is restored, place the casualty in the RECOVERY POSITION (page 41).

Even after recovery, be prepared to recommence either form of resuscitation if breathing or the heart fail again. The casualty must be removed to hospital as fast as possible after either incident.

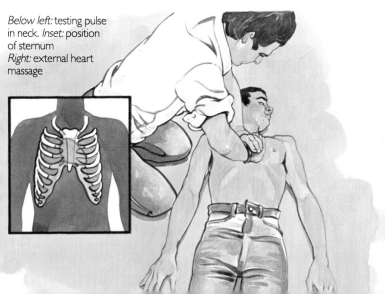

Below left: testing pulse in neck. *Inset:* position of sternum
Right: external heart massage

Bleeding (or Haemorrhage)

In external bleeding, the blood escapes from the body via a cut or other visible wound and the need for medical attention is quickly evident. Internal bleeding however, may not be apparent until a dangerous amount of blood has been lost. It may be noticed when blood is coughed up, or passed in the urine or stools. More dangerously, blood may remain concealed within the body.

The body has its own resources for stopping bleeding. Blood clots as it leaves a damaged blood vessel, the vessel contracts to reduce blood flow, and the blood pressure drops. All these measures tend to stop bleeding spontaneously, but sometimes dangerous or potentially fatal blood loss occurs before they can work.

An adult can lose a pint of blood without ill-effect, provided this is carefully taken at a blood donor session. Children can afford to lose very much less. The greater the blood loss, the greater is the threat to life. So immediate action to stop the bleeding is necessary in all but the most trivial wounds, for which only simple first aid measures are needed while the blood clots (see CUTS AND GRAZES, page 70).

Signs of excessive blood loss or concealed internal bleeding
1. Pale skin.
2. Coldness, especially of hands and feet.
3. Rapid but weak pulse – 100 beats per minute or more (this can be felt at the wrist with the finger tips).
4. Sickness and thirst.
5. Shallow breathing, gasping for air.

Your aim is to stop blood loss as soon as possible and to obtain urgent medical attention. Call 999 for Ambulance Service.

Serious external bleeding
Make the casualty lie down and, if possible, raise the injured part and keep it at rest. This allows blood to drain back into the body, and gives a blood clot chance to form without disturbance.

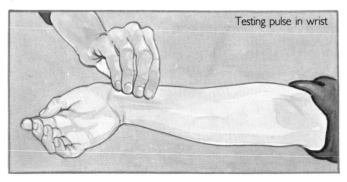

Testing pulse in wrist

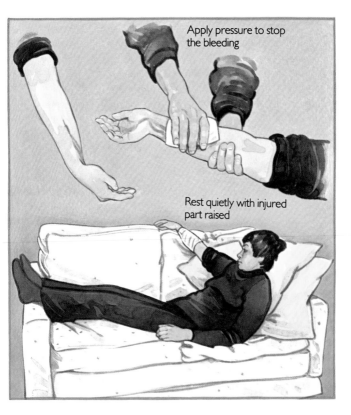

Apply pressure to stop the bleeding

Rest quietly with injured part raised

Apply pressure to the wound, preferably with a sterile dressing. If no dressing is available, and the wound is bleeding badly, use any clean material or even your hand or fingers to apply pressure until a proper dressing can be applied. If the wound is very large, press its edges together with the fingers and hold them in place until help arrives, or a clot has begun to form – this takes about 10 minutes.

Once the bleeding stops, carefully remove any dirt or surrounding foreign bodies, *but only if this can be done without the need for probing the wound.*

If you have to leave a foreign body embedded in, or protruding from the wound, put a sterile padding of gauze (*do not* use cotton wool) round the wound before applying a clean dressing, to prevent direct pressure. Hold the dressing in place with a firm bandage.

If blood soaks through the dressing, apply more dressings on top. **Do not** disturb the original dressing as to do so might dislodge the developing blood clot.

If treating a scalp wound, there may be an underlying fracture, so **do not** apply direct pressure. Apply a sterile dressing much larger than the wound, puckering the dressing at the centre to raise it clear of the wound, then circle this with a large ring pad to prevent pressure and bandage firmly in position.

Keep the casualty still and give reassurance. When the bleeding stops, get him to hospital, provided you can do this without disturbing the wound. If the bleeding shows no sign of stopping after first aid, or if blood loss is considerable, call the doctor or an ambulance immediately.

Internal bleeding

Internal blood loss can follow a fall, blow or certain medical conditions. It can be very dangerous, so get the patient to hospital as quickly as possible.

While this is being arranged, help control the bleeding by getting the casualty to lie down and rest. Raise the legs on a chair or any other convenient object, to improve the blood supply to the brain and heart.

Keep the casualty warm and comfortable, give reassurance and treat any obvious external wounds.

Do not give the casualty anything to drink or eat.

The casualty must be removed to hospital as fast as possible.

Shock

In any accident, the casualty may suffer shock. The symptoms are:
1. Cold, clammy skin.
2. Extreme pallor.
3. Sickness and giddiness.
4. Fast but shallow pulse and breathing.
5. Confusion or restlessness.

Shock casualties may gradually lose consciousness and enter into a coma. Call for medical help urgently and, while waiting for this to arrive, do what you can to make the casualty comfortable:

If he is conscious, reduce the strain on his blood circulation by lying him down. Raise the lower limbs slightly and if there is a possibility of injury to the head, chest or abdomen, prop up his head and shoulders, with his head turned to one side.

If he vomits, or loses consciousness, turn him into the RECOVERY POSITION (page 41).

Loosen any restrictive clothing, but keep him warm with extra cover, such as a blanket or coat. *Do not* use any artificial source of heat e.g. hot-water bottles.

Be prepared to give ARTIFICIAL RESPIRATION (page 44) if breathing fails.

Do not give drinks, even if the casualty complains of thirst. Simply moisten his lips with water.

3: A–Z of First Aid Treatment

Abdominal pain

Pain in the abdomen sometimes follows falls, slips or violent exertion. It is usually caused by minor tears or stretching of the sheets of muscle covering the abdomen – uncomfortable, but of little consequence unless the pain is serious enough to be inconvenient or worrying. Rest is the only cure.

The most common cause of abdominal pain is trapped gas, or "wind" in the intestine. Usually the pain clears rapidly, as the gas gurgles along the intestine. There is no real treatment, other than avoiding foods that you know cause this problem, and chewing slowly.

Other similar abdominal pains are caused by constipation. Don't take medicines to prevent constipation unless these are prescribed by the doctor. Eventually, over-use of laxatives will worsen the problem. Instead, try a high fibre diet containing wholemeal flour, or add bran to your food, and eat plenty of fruit and vegetables. If you *do* become seriously constipated, try a hot bath, and if this fails, consult your doctor.

Periods often cause abdominal pain, and most women learn to cope with this problem in their own way. In adolescent girls, period pains can be acute and very distressing. Warm baths help relaxation, together with ordinary aspirin to relieve the pain.

Pain in the abdomen after a road accident or any heavy blow to the stomach can be serious, and should receive immediate medical attention. Similarly, any persistent abdominal pain must be reported to your doctor.

Allergies

Allergic reactions happen when the body over-reacts while defending itself against something which is actually quite harmless. Grass pollen is the most common of these substances, called allergens, but there are very many others.

Hay fever, usually caused by pollen, is a summer condition, but related allergies can occur at any time of year. In an acute hay fever attack, the eyes usually become inflamed, and the nose runs, or there may be acute nasal itching, causing uncontrollable sneezing. Your doctor will probably prescribe antihistamines; if he does, be very careful about driving or operating any machine which could cause injury.

Antihistamines make most people sleepy, or slow them down considerably.

Temporary relief can be obtained by using a decongestant nasal spray which shrinks and soothes the inflamed lining of the nose. Use the spray only for the length of time specified in the instructions, or by the doctor; otherwise it may cause worse inflammation and itching. Strong light usually makes all the symptoms worse, so wear sunglasses whenever you have an attack.

Certain foods cause allergies, and the symptoms are quite different from those of hay fever. Usually food allergies cause rashes, or itchy red patches on the limbs and abdomen, or sometimes around the lips. Less commonly, food allergies cause migraines and are suspected of being involved in several quite serious illnesses. If you think you have a food allergy, try avoiding the suspect food. Common food allergens are eggs, chocolate, and strawberries. If you do identify such an allergen, let your doctor know so that it can be noted on your medical record.

Other forms of allergy are caused by skin contact. An allergy to soap powder may cause rashes due to soap remaining in incompletely rinsed clothes, for example. Some metals used in jewellery cause an allergic reaction. This is quite common with earrings and bracelets, which can leave an inflamed mark which is exactly the shape of the piece of jewellery. Don't persist in wearing the jewellery, as it could lead to more unpleasant skin conditions. Obtain an antihistamine cream from the chemist to soothe the rash.

If an allergy causes you frequent problems, consult your doctor, who may refer you to a specialised allergy clinic.

Allergies to insect bites can be dangerous, and need medical advice (see INSECT BITES).

Animal Bites

In Britain, animal bites seldom cause serious problems. Throughout most of the rest of the world, however, bites by dogs and cats in particular need immediate medical attention to eliminate the possibility of rabies infection.

Dog bites can usually be treated as "dirty" wounds. It is important not to get more dirt into the wound as you clean around it. Wipe away obvious dirt with a clean rag or tissue, cleaning *away* from the bite. Gradually clean in towards the wound, still wiping *away*.

Once superficial dirt is removed, clean the bite thoroughly under cold running water, or water containing properly diluted medical disinfectant (follow the instructions on the label). The wound should soon stop bleeding. Dry the whole area of skin around the bite with clean tissue or cotton wool, and apply an adhesive plaster – but *not* the waterproof type.

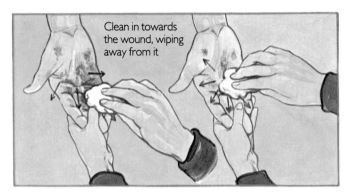

Clean in towards the wound, wiping away from it

Contact your doctor for advice. If the bite was deep, an anti-tetanus "shot" may be necessary, and if there is a risk of other types of infection, antibiotics may be needed.

Bites and scratches from cats are not usually deep, and do not normally need further treatment after cleaning up.

Small pets like hamsters and rabbits can give very deep and painful bites, which may need further medical treatment after cleaning and covering the wound.

Bites from any wild animal may carry a risk of infection, and you should seek medical advice without delay.
☐See also INSECT BITES and SNAKE BITES.

Assault and Rape

When a person has been assaulted there may be any of a number of injuries. Examine the casualty quickly to see what first aid measures are needed, and act accordingly, referring to the relevant entries in this A–Z. At least as important is the emotional effect on an assaulted person. They will need reassurance and comfort as much as first aid. Usually they will be worried about contacting other members of their family, so get from them a telephone number or address as quickly as possible. Telephone the police, so that they can take over but offer to stay with the casualty. A friendly presence can be very comforting.

In any assault or rape there will probably be legal repercussions, and it is very important to bear this in mind. Unfortunately, it means that the casualty must not be cleaned up before the police arrive, as otherwise important evidence could be destroyed. Obviously, essential first aid must be carried out, such as wound dressing, or any measures necessary to protect life. Retain any of the casualties clothing that you *have to* remove for first aid, as the police will want to examine it.
☐See especially BLEEDING, BROKEN BONES AND DISLOCATIONS, FAINTING, HEAD INJURIES AND CONCUSSION, HYSTERIA, and PENETRATING WOUNDS.

Asthmatic Attacks

Over a million people in Britain suffer from asthma, and many of them experience attacks in which breathing becomes seriously restricted by contraction of air tubes in the lungs. Such attacks can be caused by an allergy (see ALLERGIES, page 51), emotional or physical stress, or less obvious factors.

Most asthmatics carry tablets or inhalers which relieve the wheezing very rapidly if an attack develops. If they have a serious attack, however, they may need your help in locating and giving them their emergency treatment.

First attacks, especially in children, are very alarming, both for the child and the parent. And none of the special drugs will be available to ease the attack.

Loosen the casualty's clothing to allow easier breathing, and either sit him up or get him to stand, leaning forward slightly.

This allows the chest to be expanded more effectively during breathing.

Try to calm and reassure the patient. Panicky overbreathing only makes the symptoms worse.

If it is a first attack, contact the doctor immediately. If the casualty takes anti-asthmatic drugs, or uses an inhaler, the attack should subside quickly.

Watch the patient carefully, and if, in spite of drug treatment or use of an inhaler, the symptoms seem to be getting steadily worse, contact the doctor quickly.

There are breathing exercises designed to help asthmatics to clear air from the lungs and strengthen the muscles used in breathing. Details of these exercises can be obtained from your doctor, or a local asthma or allergy clinic. A special booklet on breathing exercises is available direct from the Asthma Research Council, 12 Pembridge Square, London W2 4EM. Ask the doctor about literature describing ways to make asthma attacks less likely e.g. by frequent changes of bed linen and dust prevention.

Two positions to ease asthmatic attacks

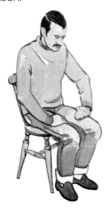

Back and Neck Injuries

The spinal cord runs through a series of bony rings called vertebrae, which are jointed to allow the whole spine to bend. If the spine is bent too far, however, one or more vertebrae may shatter, and sometimes sections of splintered bone damage the spinal cord itself.

Fracture of the spine, including the neck, is therefore a very dangerous injury. It may be a sports injury, such as when a high diver hits the bottom of the pool, or a rugby scrum collapses. Falls from a considerable height, or from a motor bike, can also cause spinal injuries. In motor accidents, when a car is struck from behind or head on, whiplash injuries of the neck can be sustained.

If there is the slightest suspicion of damage to the spine, **do not** move the casualty at all. Movement could cause already damaged vertebrae to splinter further and affect the spinal cord. Sitting the casualty up is the worst thing you could do. Keep him flat, and if help is a long while arriving, cover him with a coat or blanket to prevent chilling.

You can test for damage to the spinal cord by making sure the casualty can move fingers and toes, and has no loss of sensation, or complains of "pins and needles" in the fingers or toes.

While waiting for qualified first-aiders or an ambulance crew to arrive, prevent the casualty from trying to move himself (with risk of further damage). If necessary, tie ankles and knees loosely together to immobilise the legs.

A very common back injury, generally incorrectly referred to as "slipped disc", often occurs while bending, or straining to lift a heavy object. This can be very frightening, as it is often too painful to move at all, and it may take a long while to get the casualty safely indoors or to a doctor.

This type of back injury happens when nerves running out between the bony vertebrae get pinched by over-movement of the spine. Depending on which nerves are affected, this may cause pain, loss of sensation, or both. Similar injuries happen when a ligament in the spine is torn or stretched. Because the lower spine is most liable to such damage, the area around the hips and legs is most often affected.

Get the casualty indoors, and lying flat. Give painkillers like aspirin or paracetamol, and call the doctor to make sure there is no serious damage. A special hard bed, or a board under the mattress may help prevent the trouble recurring. Ask the doctor for detailed advice.

A true "slipped disc" is more serious, but quite rare. It happens when the cushion of rubbery cartilage between the vertebrae bursts under a heavy load. Portions of the damaged cartilage may press on the spinal cord, but even if this does not happen, the condition is very painful and needs prolonged specialist treatment.

You will not be able to tell "slipped disc" from lesser back problems, until it has been properly diagnosed by the doctor.

Torn or "pulled" muscles in the back, caused by falls, or by sudden twists, usually while carrying heavy loads are very common and painful, but not at all dangerous. These, too, are treated by immobilisation in bed, plenty of rest, and painkillers.

Bandaging and Wound Dressing

In first aid, bandages may be applied for any of several purposes:
1. To control bleeding.
2. To keep a dressing in place over a wound.
3. To reduce risk of wound infection.
4. To prevent further injury.
5. To prevent movement.

Bandages can be improvised in an emergency from any clean fabric, such as a shirt, sheet, or tablecloth. Many first aid kits include specially made triangular bandages which can be used for a variety of purposes, but these are difficult to apply without specialised first aid training. More useful in the home is the roller bandage – a long gauze or cloth strip available in a range of widths. It is supplied pre-packed and rolled, and can be purchased sterile. Elasticated roller bandages are also available to support injured parts such as

sprained wrists or ankles.

Dressings are used to cover a wound. Most useful in the home are adhesive dressings, generally known as "plasters". These consist of an adhesive backing, to which is attached an absorbent pad, which helps to dry up fluids seeping from the wound. The backing may be made from various fabrics or plastic materials. Ideally, the dressings should be porous, or perforated, to prevent perspiration from building up underneath, reducing adhesion.

Adhesive dressings will stick well only on dry skin. They should be used only on small wounds, or after heavy bleeding has stopped.

Dressings tend to adhere to wounds as the blood and secretions dry. This can happen with adhesive dressings, or with loose gauze dressings, which are simply laid over a wound and held on with bandages or adhesive plaster.

Special non-stick dressings with a perforated plastic film covering are available, and these will peel off easily, without causing pain, when they have to be removed.

All dressings applied to an open wound should be sterile. They usually come packed in sealed paper sachets, which are only removed immediately before use. Wash your hands before handling them, and make sure that your fingers do not touch the part of the dressing which will be in direct contact with the wound.

Always use a dressing of adequate size to absorb blood or secretions which would otherwise soon penetrate, and make a change of both dressing and bandage necessary.

If a dressing sticks to the wound when you try to remove it, soak the affected part in warm water to loosen it.

To remove from the skin sticky marks left by adhesive dressings or plaster bandages, use special solvent available from your chemist.

Bandaging holds a loose dressing firmly in place (take care not to dislodge the dressing as you begin bandaging); this must be tight enough to ensure that the dressing cannot shift, but must never be so tight as to reduce the circulation. Signs of a too-tight bandage are numbness or whiteness of fingers or toes.

When using a roller bandage, it is important to match its width to the job it is to do. For hands and fingers, narrow bandages of 2.5–5 cm (1–2 inch) width are necessary. For arms and legs, 5 to 8.5 cm (2–3½ inch) wide bandages are suitable, and for bandaging the trunk, even wider.

Bandages must be applied under tension. They are kept rolled, with the loose end being applied to the wounded part. First a loose loop is made around the injured part, and a light pull is given to the rolled bandage to secure it. The *outer* surface of the rolled bandage is applied to the skin.

Then the rolled bandage is passed round and round the injured part in a spiral, overlapping each previous turn by about two-thirds. Keep steady tension on the bandage as it is applied.

Sometimes several layers of bandage are needed for security, spiralling along then reversing direction. Complete the bandaging by making a final straight turn above the injury, doubling the end over, and securing it with a safety pin or strip of adhesive plaster.

To ensure that bandages on limbs stay in place, start nearest the foot or hand, and work inwards towards the body. If the bandage covers the knee or elbow, pass the bandage around the limb, first above, then below the joint to ensure that it is not dislodged as the limb flexes.

Allowance has to be made for awkward shapes, such as the thumb, when bandaging the hand. Usually by spiralling the bandage above and below the thumb, or any other obstruction, the wound can be securely covered.

If the bandage tends to slip off, as when bandaging the thigh or upper arm, apply in a figure-of-eight pattern. This grips better and remains secure.

In any difficult area, elasticated crêpe bandages remain in place more securely.

Bandages (roller or triangular) can also be used as slings (see BROKEN BONES AND DISLOCATIONS, page 61).

Some of the bandaging techniques mentioned are illustrated on pages 58–59.

Below: three steps to making a ring pad from roller bandage.
Right: applying adhesive dressing.
Below right: apply bandage of appropriate width, under tension, overlapping by about two-thirds. For elbow, pass bandage around limb, first above then below joint to make it really secure.
Far right, top: allow for awkward shapes, such as thumbs by spiralling bandage above and below thumb, as shown.
Far right, centre: bandage should hold dressing firmly, but not so tightly that circulation is affected.
Far right, below: roller bandage applied in a figure-of-eight

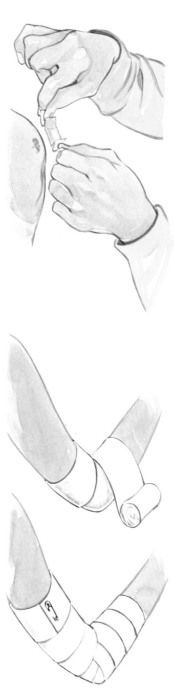

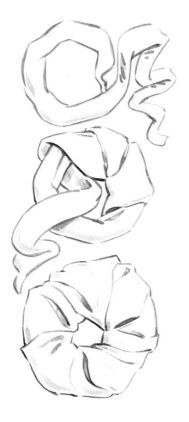

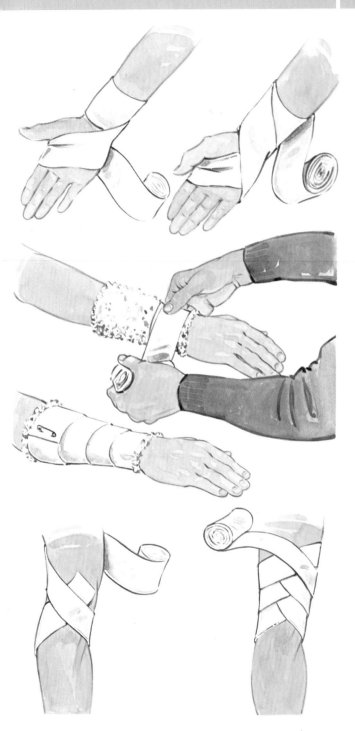

Bites and Stings

Different types of bites and stings are treated under separate headings in this book. Apart from immediate pain, damage, and discomfort caused by any bite or sting, always bear in mind the possiblity of later infection. If there is painful swelling around a bite or sting, and it appears to be getting worse, obtain proper treatment from your doctor without delay. □See also ANIMAL BITES, HOLIDAY PROBLEMS, INSECT BITES, SNAKE BITES.

Black Eye

The swelling and discolouration of a black eye are the result of bruising. Minor internal bleeding into the tissues causes swelling around the eyelid, partly closing the eye.

The only treatment is an ice-pack; applied to the eye as soon as possible after the injury. For details, see BRUISING (page 66). Once swelling and discolouration has appeared, nothing more can be done to treat the black eye. The application of the traditional piece of steak to the eye is useless.

The eye is a very delicate organ. Any blow serious enough to cause a black eye could possibly cause eye damage, or even a fractured skull. Have it seen by your doctor as soon as possible to make sure there is no serious damage.

Bleeding (or Haemorrhage) see page 48

Blisters

Blisters are fluid-filled bubbles formed when the top layer of skin separates from the tissues beneath, as a result of continuous rubbing of the skin, or from a burn.

The fluid in the blister will eventually be absorbed again, leaving the dry outer layer of skin to peel away. Sometimes the blister breaks spontaneously, hastening its healing. Only if the blister is a serious inconvenience, or is liable to be further rubbed and irritated by the clothing or by shoes, should it be *carefully* pricked with a sterilised needle to release the fluid. To prevent infection, first wash the blister and surrounding skin with soap and water, followed by antiseptic diluted exactly as instructed on the label. Heat a large sewing needle in a gas flame until the tip is red hot, then hold the needle for a few minutes until the tip has cooled, being careful not to let it touch anything else.

Prick the blister at two or more points around its base (this will be painless). Press gently with a wad of clean cotton wool to expel the clear fluid in the blister, then cover the whole area with an adhesive dressing for a few days. If there is any pain or inflammation in the area around the blister, *do not* attempt to prick it. The blister may be infected, and your doctor should be consulted.

Breathing Problems see page 42

Broken Bones and Dislocations

A broken or fractured bone may break clean across, crack, or be completely shattered. In a very bad break, broken ends of the bone can penetrate through the skin, with a risk of later infection.

In a dislocation, a joint becomes wrenched so badly that bones leave their sockets. The symptoms are usually similar to a broken bone.

In some accidents, due to the unnatural limb position, it is obvious that a bone has broken, as it is also when broken bone penetrates through the skin.

Sometimes, however, it is not so easy to tell if there is an actual break. Below are several possible signs and symptoms of a break:

1. The casualty may have felt, or heard, the bone snap, or may be able to describe the accident in such a way that there is no doubt about its result.

2. Pain at or near the site of the break will be very severe. Movement of the affected part will be difficult or impossible.
3. The whole area will be extremely tender to the touch.
4. There may be a deformity or abnormality, such as twisting or bending of a broken limb.
5. The area of the break will swell rapidly, due to bleeding into the tissues.
6. Movement may appear unnatural, if possible at all. The casualty may feel a grating sensation in the damaged part.

There are several important aims of first aid in the event of broken bones. Treat other serious injuries such as bleeding, breathing difficulties or severe wounds before dealing with the fracture.

Fractures where broken bones have penetrated the skin should be covered immediately. Do not attempt to clean such wounds yourself, or touch them with your fingers. Cover them with a sterile dressing, or if this is not available, with any clean material.

Immobilise or support the damaged part so that no further injury occurs. Do not attempt to straighten or move the injured parts, and avoid all unnecessary movement of the casualty. If it is absolutely essential to move a broken limb, because the casualty's position makes further injury likely, you will have to apply traction to avoid pain and damage. Pull the limb gently but firmly away from the body, gripping either hand or foot.

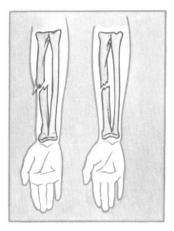

Open fracture and closed fracture

Manoeuvre the limb carefully to a more comfortable position, keeping up the traction all the time. Release the limb gradually to avoid causing more pain.

Call an ambulance in all but minor breaks. In lesser injuries, such as a broken wrist, it is usually possible to take the casualty to hospital by car.

You will have to immobilise the injured part as soon as possible. A broken leg is best immobilised by tying or bandaging it to the other uninjured leg. If both legs are broken, splints have to be used.

Arms are easily immobilised by tying them to the side or chest.

Many specialised first aid techniques are available for immobilising or splinting broken bones, but in most domestic accidents, the following simple measures are usually adequate.

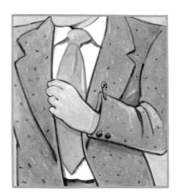

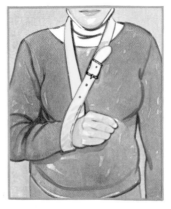

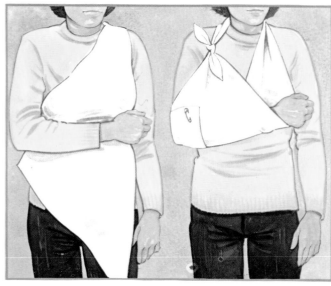

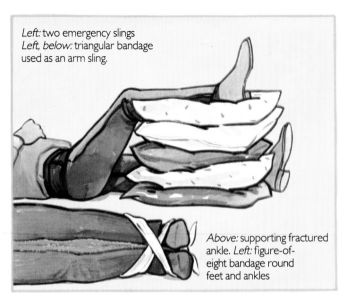

Left: two emergency slings
Left, below: triangular bandage used as an arm sling.

Above: supporting fractured ankle. *Left:* figure-of-eight bandage round feet and ankles

Broken arms: in breaks to the upper arms, or to the bones of the shoulder, the casualty usually eases the pain naturally by taking the weight of the elbow in the other hand, hugging the broken arm against his side. This actually immobilises the break very effectively, and is sometimes sufficient while you get the casualty to hospital by car.

A sling can be applied to give better support. This will definitely be needed if the break is lower down in the forearm.

Breaks in the elbow region can cause great damage to blood vessels, and in this instance the broken arm **must be kept straight**. Tie the arm loosely to the side of the body, or lie it extended by the side on a pillow and wait for help to arrive.

Broken legs: a broken leg is very serious, as heavy internal bleeding can occur. The leg must be immobilised by bringing the good leg around carefully to lie alongside the damaged one. Use folded clothing to pad between the legs, especially the knees, then tie ankles and knees firmly together with bandages (but not so tight as to cut off blood circulation). Tie wide bandages above and below the break, tightening them very cautiously. Make no further attempt to move the casualty yourself. If bandages are not available, improvise with scarves, ties or belts.

In broken ankles, feet, or toes, **do not** remove footwear, as this helps support the damaged part. First aid involves simply keeping all weight off the break, so you may sometimes be able to get the casualty to hospital yourself, by car. If you cannot transport the casualty to hospital, raise the leg and make it comfortable on a pile of cushions.

In a very serious accident, where both legs are broken, you must call an ambulance immediately, before attempting first aid. Try to straighten the limbs very gradually, using traction. Tie the ankles loosely together. Pad between the legs and immobilise the limbs, by tying any suitable long objects like walking sticks or umbrellas along the side of the legs and the trunk. Try to pass the bandages under the body at points where it does not involve moving the casualty too much, e.g. under the ankles, knees, and above and below the buttocks.

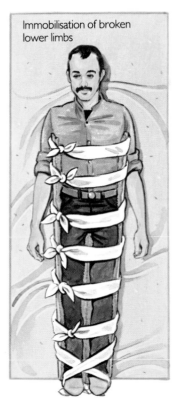

Immobilisation of broken lower limbs

Spinal injuries: first aid treatment for a broken spine consists of immobilisation, and immediate expert help.

If a broken neck is suspected, the head must be immobilised **without moving it in any way**. This can be done by making a collar from a rolled-up newspaper, and gently, carefully tying it around the neck with a bandage, steadying the head as you do so to prevent it rolling to one side.

Broken ribs: if a rib is broken, there will be very sharp pains in the chest. The casualty takes shallow breaths because of the pain. If the broken rib has punctured a lung, blood will be coughed up. In a very bad break, there may be an open wound to the chest, which allows air to be sucked in. This must be sealed immediately, preferably with an adhesive plaster dressing, or otherwise by covering with any suitable clean material, held securely in place by hand or by firm bandaging.

If the casualty is conscious, prop him up in a comfortable sitting position, or leaning over *towards the injured side.* If unconscious, lay him on his injured side, with head slightly down.

Dislocations: a dislocation is a joint injury, and sometimes occurs together with a break. It is often difficult to distinguish from a broken bone.

The symptoms are very similar, except that a dislocation always occurs at a joint, causing it to be unnaturally fixed whereas

A newspaper, folded as shown makes an effective emergency collar to support neck; carefully overlap the curved ends round the back of the neck and hold in position with a handkerchief, a tie, a scarf or a piece of string tied round the "collar"

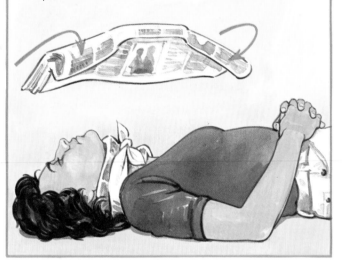

a broken bone is unnaturally mobile at the site of the fracture. However, the pain is such that the casualty will seldom even attempt to move, often feeling very sick.

As with a break, first aid treatment is to support the injured part. **Never** attempt to replace the bones in their normal position. Support injured parts on a pillow or pad, or immobilise them firmly as described above for broken bones. Keep a close watch for signs that circulation is affected, such as whiteness of fingers or toes, or loss of sensation. If this occurs, straighten the limb very gently, but **do not** use traction. ☐See also BACK INJURIES, HEAD INJURIES, FINGER AND TOE INJURIES, and SPLINTS.

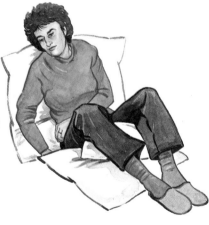

A conscious casualty with chest injuries should be supported in a half-sitting position

Bruises

A bruise is the result of a blow to the body which causes bleeding beneath the skin, usually without actually breaking the skin. Blood filtering out of damaged blood vessels causes swelling and discolouration, and the whole area will be tender to the touch for some time.

Medical help is not usually needed, except to confirm that there are no less apparent injuries.

Once the bruise has appeared, nothing can be done to hasten its clearance. You can reduce the likelihood of a bruise, by treating the injured part yourself immediately after an accident.

Raise the injured part to reduce the amount of blood present.

Apply a cold compress of towelling or other material, soaked in cold water, to the injury, replacing the compress periodically with further cold, soaked material.

Alternatively, prepare an ice pack by putting ice cubes and table salt in a polythene bag. Tie the neck of the bag in a secure knot, roll it in a towel, and apply to the wound.

Keep up the cold treatment for an hour. After that, any bruises will have formed and there is no point in further treatment.
☐See also BLACK EYE.

Burns and scalds

Burns are among the most serious of common accidents.

Only the smallest burns can be safely treated by yourself – with any large burn there is a risk of scarring, infection and sometimes, risk to life. If in doubt, always get medical attention as quickly as possible.

There is no real difference between burns and scalds. Burns are caused by contact with hot objects, chemicals, electricity or friction, while scalds are caused by contact with boiling liquids or by steam.

In any burn or scald, your first objective is to reduce the immediate effects of the heat, by cooling the injured part.

Cool the injury under a cold running tap, or immerse it in water, and keep it there for at least 10 minutes, except in the most minor burns. This greatly reduces the extent of the injury, and reduces the amount of medical treatment which will be needed.

In chemical burns, use the same technique of washing the injured area with cold water for at least 10 minutes. If the eyes are affected, gently separate the eyelids between fingers and thumb, and bathe the eyeball thoroughly but with care (see page 74).

In electrical burns, proceed in the same way, but first make absolutely sure that the electrical power supply is no longer a hazard before using any water (see ELECTRIC SHOCK page 34).

With a scald, or chemical burn, remove clothing soaked in hot liquids. If clothes are charred by fire, **do not** attempt to remove them; leave this for trained staff at the hospital.

Remove shoes, watches, or jewellery which might cut into the skin as injured parts begin to swell.

Under no circumstances should you apply grease, ointment, or antiseptic to any burned parts. **Do not** touch the injury with cotton wool or any fluffy material which could stick to the wound.

Lay the casualty down, and cover the burned part with clean, non-linty material, such as bed linen. **Do not** let the casualty move about while waiting for medical help to arrive.

Give a *conscious* casualty small amounts of a cold drink at frequent intervals, but **do not** give alcohol. Drinks help to replace lost body fluid. **Never** attempt to give drinks to an unconscious casualty. This could cause vomiting and possible choking.

Even small burns and scalds can leave scars, and only small shallow burns of up to 1 cm (½ inch) diameter should be treated at home. Clean the injury thoroughly using water, and cover with a plaster or a dressing and bandage. Relieve pain from these minor burns with ordinary aspirin or paracetamol following the dosage instructions on the pack. □See also ELECTRIC SHOCK, LIGHTNING, and SUNBURN.

Childbirth (emergency) see page 37

Chilling and Hypothermia

Continuous exposure to low temperatures can lead to a dangerous drop in body temperature in the elderly or the very young.

Old people do not generate body heat so efficiently, and may not be able to afford to heat their home adequately. Babies lose heat very quickly if, for example, they are insufficiently clothed in a cold room. Both the old and the very young may gradually slide into a stupor and unconsciousness.

When body temperature drops below 35°C (95°F), a state of hypothermia occurs.
In babies, the symptoms are sometimes confusing. They first become subdued and lose their appetite as their temperature falls, and the skin of their chest feels cold – but their skin may become red. Immediate medical attention is required. If possible, get the baby to hospital without delay. If this is not possible, remove the baby's clothing and get into bed with him, using skin-to-skin contact to warm him *gradually*.
Adults, and especially the elderly, become very pale and sometimes the skin appears bluish in colour. Breathing becomes very shallow and the pulse is extremely weak.

First aid measures are aimed at preventing further heat loss, then *gradually* improving body temperature.

Wrap the casualty in blankets and warm clothes and, if they are conscious, give sips of warm drinks. **Do not** try to warm them up with hot water bottles, electric blankets, or hot baths. The sudden surge of blood into newly warmed tissues would drain blood from the heart and other vital organs, and could even lead to heart failure.

Get the casualty to hospital as soon as possible, or call the doctor.

□See also EXPOSURE.

Choking

Choking is caused by any obstruction of the air passages to the lungs.

In minor choking, as when a drink "goes down the wrong way", there is usually little to be done but watch the choking person to make sure that the coughing and spluttering does not get worse. The body attempts to dislodge or eject anything passing into the lungs or air passages, and coughing is the natural defensive reflex.

In true choking, the lungs become blocked off completely by whatever was inhaled. The casualty rapidly becomes blue, and loses consciousness. You may be able to hook out the obstruction from the mouth, using your finger, but it may have been inhaled more deeply and be out of reach.

In this case, swiftly give a series of hard blows between the shoulders. Depending on age, position the casualty as follows:

Babies: hold them upside-down by the ankles, and slap them between the shoulders

Children: lay them face down over the knee, and slap the back hard

Adults: get the casualty to lean

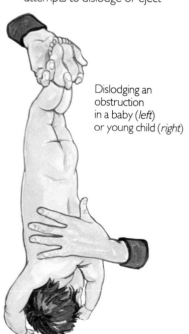

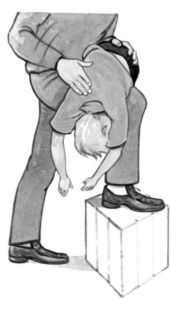

Dislodging an obstruction in a baby (*left*) or young child (*right*)

over the back of a chair so that his head is lower than his chest and strike hard between his shoulders, using the flat of the hand.

If casualty remains limp or blue, or if he does not seem to be breathing properly, follow with ARTIFICIAL RESPIRATION (page 44) or HEART MASSAGE (page 46). Even if the blockage remains you may be able to blow life-saving air past it.

Convulsions

Convulsions or fits are uncontrollable spasms of the muscles, together with loss of consciousness, twitching, and rolling of the eyes.

In adults or adolescents, they are usually caused by EPILEPSY (page 72) or by overdoses of DRUGS (page 72), but in babies, a fever or HEAT STROKE (page 79) can also cause convulsions.

In a baby with a convulsion, the face may twitch, eyes roll or cross, and the body arches backwards, usually with the breath held. The face becomes red and congested, and frothy spittle may appear in the mouth.

There is no effective treatment, and you must **never** attempt to force the mouth open, or restrain the limbs, except to move the convulsing casualty clear of any object on which they might injure themselves, and stay with them.

Loosen tight clothing to ensure a good air supply. When the convulsion has passed, lay the casualty in the RECOVERY POSITION (page 41).

If a baby has a very high temperature, sponge him with tepid water to bring it down. Allow the water to dry on the skin.

Call the doctor as soon as possible.
☐See also EPILEPSY, DRUGS and HEAT STROKE.

Cramp

Cramp is a sudden, uncontrollable contraction of a muscle, or group of muscles. It can be caused by chilling, extreme muscular fatigue, or by loss of salt or fluids from the body after excessive sweating, diarrhoea, or vomiting. In the latter case, treat by giving large quantities of water to drink, to which is added ½ teaspoonful of table salt per 600 ml (1 pint).

In the more common cramps following exertion or chilling, relief can be obtained by forcibly straightening the cramped limb and, when the muscle relaxes, massaging it vigorously.

Crushing, Injuries due to

Injuries may range from fingers pinched by a closing door to extensive injuries to large parts of the body caused by motor accidents.

Frequently, there is little visible injury but soft tissues such as muscle and skin are damaged, and there will be considerable swelling due to blood and other fluids escaping from damaged vessels.

For most minor crush injuries, apply a cold compress (see BRUISES, page 66).

In more serious injuries, raise the injured part to reduce the leakage of fluids, and bind firmly with a crêpe or elastic bandage.

In extensive crushing, internal injury may be serious. Lay the casualty flat with the legs raised. Call for medical help urgently.

While waiting for help to arrive keep the casualty warm. Give sips of cold water *only* if there is no reason to suspect internal abdominal damage.
☐See also BREATHING PROBLEMS.

Cuts and Grazes

Small cuts and shallow grazes seldom cause serious medical problems. They can be treated successfully at home. However, large, ragged, or dirty injuries need proper medical treatment including, possibly, an anti-tetanus injection.

When treating a cut or graze, first clean your own hands thoroughly.

Remove any obvious dirt, gravel, or metal. Then thoroughly clean the skin around the wound, using gauze or cotton wool moistened with water or properly diluted disinfectant. Cleanse *away* from the wound to prevent more dirt from being introduced.

Small wounds can be washed directly under running water.

Dry the wound carefully, and apply a dressing (see BANDAGING AND WOUND DRESSING, page 56). **Do not** put antiseptic cream on the injury, as this only seals in dirt and germs. The wound should soon stop

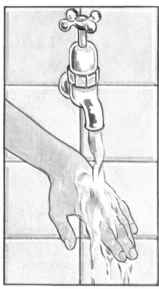
Washing a small wound

bleeding of its own accord as the blood clots. If not, treat as described under BLEEDING (page 48).

When the wound has dried, remove the dressing, to hasten the healing process.

Any wound which continues to weep or ooze fluid, bleeds excessively, or becomes sore and inflamed, should be seen by your doctor.
☐See also BANDAGING AND WOUND DRESSING, and BLEEDING.

Dehydration see HEAT STROKE, page 79.

Diabetes

Diabetes results from a fault in the normal usage of sugar, which fuels the body. It arises because of a deficiency of an enzyme called insulin, which has to be supplemented by frequent insulin injections, or the use of other drugs.

Most people with diabetes know the dangers, and can avoid them, but sometimes first aid measures are needed.

Two serious conditions can affect the diabetic:

Too much insulin/too little sugar: sometimes a diabetic patient under treatment has too much insulin in the bloodstream. This may be due to accidental overdosing, or the balance of insulin and sugar may have been disturbed by missing a meal, or by burning up too much sugar by over-exertion.

This condition usually comes on slowly, but the diabetic patient may not notice the symptoms: paleness, sweating, trembling, rapid shallow breathing, and confusion. Sometimes the diabetic appears to be aggressively drunk. Fainting, coma, even death may follow if the diabetic does not receive prompt medical attention to build up blood sugar levels.

Too little insulin/too much sugar: if the diabetic forgets to take his insulin, he may gradually slip into a deep coma, with flushed face, a dry skin and very deep, slow breathing. The breath has a characteristic smell rather like nail varnish remover.

If the casualty is conscious, and confirms that he is diabetic, give him large amounts of sugar in the quickest possible way – as sugar lumps, sweet drinks, or any sweet foods.

Most diabetics carry a supply of sugar lumps in case of such emergencies. If he recovers very quickly, he was suffering from too much insulin, or too little sugar. In the other form of diabetic attack, caused by lack of insulin, there will be no response.

In either case, get the casualty to hospital quickly.

If the casualty is unconscious, check his wallet or purse for a card stating that he is diabetic. Finding sugar lumps in the pocket is also a strong indication of diabetes. **Do not** attempt to force sugar down an unconscious diabetic, as this could cause vomiting.

Turn the casualty into the RECOVERY POSITION (page 41) and obtain medical assistance urgently.

Diarrhoea

Diarrhoea is a medical problem which should be treated by your doctor if it persists for more than 24 hours. In babies, copious diarrhoea should be reported to the doctor immediately.

In the short term, take a kaolin and morphine mixture or tablets obtained from the chemist, in the dosage recommended on the bottle or pack. If the condition has not improved within 24 hours, contact the doctor. Call the doctor immediately if there is blood in the diarrhoea.
☐See also FOOD POISONING, HOLIDAY PROBLEMS.

Drowning see page 36.

Drugs and Alcohol

Intoxication can occur from taking drugs or from alcohol. In either case, abnormal behaviour is caused by the effects of poisons on the brain.

If the casualty appears to be intoxicated, try to find out what he has taken. Even if a person's breath smells of alcohol, drunkenness is not necessarily the cause of his behaviour. He may have taken another type of drug, or be suffering from an illness such as EPILEPSY (page 72) or DIABETES (page 70), which can sometimes cause confusion.

If you are sure that a person is suffering from drug intoxication, call for medical assistance immediately and state which drug has caused the problem.

If you think the casualty is drunk, watch to make sure he does not appear to be getting worse. Taken in sufficient quantity, alcohol can kill.

A deeply intoxicated person can progress through confusion and stupor to unconsciousness, coma and death. Death results from failure of breathing, sometimes due to inhaled vomit. If the casualty deteriorates suddenly while you are waiting for medical assistance, be prepared to give ARTIFICIAL RESPIRATION (page 44) if necessary.

If the casualty becomes unconscious, turn him into the RECOVERY POSITION (page 41). □See also BREATHING PROBLEMS, CHOKING, UNCONSCIOUSNESS and POISONING.

Ear Injuries

The ear is prone to several types of damage.

Damage to the outer part of the ear and its lobe will cause copious bleeding, best controlled by pressure over a dressing or a piece of clean material. Maintain the pressure for at least 10 minutes, while the blood clots. Then put on a clean dressing and bandage, and have the injury seen by a doctor.

Bleeding from inside the ear canal can result from a scratch or infected spot inside the ear. Much more seriously, such bleeding can be caused by a blow or explosive blast which ruptures the eardrum. This will also cause deafness and often a temporary loss of balance.

A blow on the head, fracturing the skull, can also cause bleeding from the ear.

Never attempt to stem the flow of blood by plugging the ear, as this could cause infection. Lie the casualty down, with the injured ear tilted *downwards* to encourage drainage of the blood. Avoid touching the ear or surrounding area.

Get medical aid immediately, and keep a careful watch for deterioration in breathing. □See also HEAD INJURIES AND CONCUSSION, and FOREIGN BODIES.

Electric Shock see page 34.

Epilepsy

In minor attacks: the casualty is simply not conscious of his surroundings. He grows pale and his eyes become fixed and staring. Then he may just resume whatever he was doing, quite unaware that he has suffered a fit. Treat as for FAINTING (page 74).

In major attacks: the casualty may be forewarned by a headache, a feeling of strangeness and irritability or lethargy.

He will lose consciousness rapidly, falling to the ground and remaining rigid momentarily, then going into noisy convulsions.

He may also froth at the mouth and, if he involuntarily bites his tongue, the froth will be blood-stained.

Quickly remove from his proximity all hard objects on which he might injure himself, e.g. tables or chairs. **Do not** attempt to restrain him. **Do not** attempt to force his mouth open, but if an opportunity arises, carefully remove any dentures and place a wad of clean, soft material far back between his jaws to prevent him biting his tongue.

Wipe away any froth around his mouth.

Ease any tight clothing, then turn the casualty into the RECOVERY POSITION (page 41) and keep watch until he is fully recovered. He should then see his doctor.

Exposure

Exposure is a condition affecting people caught outdoors in cold, wet weather, while wearing unsuitable clothing. It is a condition of hypothermia (see CHILLING, page 67), where the body temperature drops to a dangerously low level, due to excess heat loss. It differs from the most common form of hypothermia, which normally affects the elderly or babies, in that healthy adolescents or adults are usually the victims, while mountaineering, caving, hiking, etcetera.

The condition develops very slowly, and the victim may not notice its effects until too late. The early symptoms are physical and mental sluggishness, cramps, and shivering. These gradually get worse, speech becomes slurred and vision blurred. The pulse rate increases at first, then both pulse and breathing rate begin to fall.

If you, or a member of your party experience any of these symptoms while on a prolonged outdoor trip, **do not** attempt to force the pace to get the casualty home.

Prevent further heat loss by shielding the casualty from the wind or rain. Cover him with a blanket, groundsheet, polythene, or anything which will act as a windbreak. Give him high energy food such as chocolate and warm drinks containing sugar. **Do not** give alcohol. Cover his face and hands as much as possible, as heat is lost from these areas.

Once you do reach home, help the casualty into a warm bath with a temperature of about 43°C (109°F). This is just about bearable to a dipped-in elbow. Support the casualty in the bath in case he loses consciousness.

When the casualty recovers, dry him thoroughly and wrap him up warmly. Get medical attention urgently, even if recovery appears to be complete.
☐See also CHILLING and FROSTBITE.

Eye Injuries

The eye is susceptible to several forms of serious damage. A violent blow causes external damage to the eyelids and surrounding tissues, resulting in a black eye. It can also damage the tiny blood vessels within the eye, the bleeding causing deterioration of vision. Penetrating wounds, caused by splinters or metal particles are especially serious, and can cause permanent damage or blindness.

If the eye is splashed with any chemical, wash it out **immediately**, with lots of water. Turn the head so that the

chemical will not be washed into the good eye. Pull the eyelid back with your fingers, and allow a gentle flow of water to run directly sideways over the eyeball, for at least 10 minutes. Use a tap or shower head. (Water should **never** be directed straight at the cornea from a tap as it could damage it.)

For any eye injury, other than a small foreign body which is easily removed, hospital treatment is urgently needed.

Close the injured eye, cover it with a soft dressing and bandage gently around the head to keep the dressing secure. Take the casualty to hospital as soon as possible – **do not** wait for the doctor or ambulance to arrive.
☐See also BLACK EYE and FOREIGN BODIES.

Fainting

Fainting occurs when the blood supply to the brain is temporarily reduced. Loss of consciousness is brief, as once the casualty is lying flat the blood supply is quickly restored.

Fainting can be brought on by a shock, fright, or exhaustion. Prolonged standing can drain blood from the brain into the legs, causing a faint. Similarly, injury or the early stages of some illnesses can cause fainting.

The casualty may have some warning, feeling dizzy and cold. The face becomes very pale as blood drains from the upper part of the body, and the casualty may break out in a cold sweat.

Sometimes the faint can be

Direct water flow with care when washing chemicals out of an eye

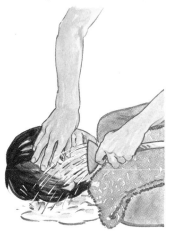

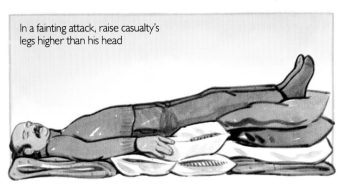

In a fainting attack, raise casualty's legs higher than his head

prevented by flexing the leg muscles to help blood circulation. Loosen clothing at the neck and waist, and sit the casualty down, with his head lowered between his knees. When he feels better, give sips of cold water.

If the casualty has passed out completely, lay him down, loosen clothing as above, and raise his legs to a higher level than his head.

Upon recovery, give him sips of water.

Treat any associated injury. Use your discretion as to whether medical treatment is necessary.

Finger and Toe Injuries

Among the most common and painful injuries are those caused by crushing a finger or toe in a door, or by dropping a heavy object on one's foot. Usually, painful bleeding under the nail results, and the nail may subsequently come off.

Holding the injured part under a cold running tap for 10 minutes, will prevent much of the swelling. Take aspirin to

reduce the pain, and consult the doctor. He may be able to save the nail by making a small (and painless) hole in it to release trapped blood.

Fish Hook Injuries

Fish hooks caught in the skin are best removed by a doctor, to avoid risk of infection. But in an emergency there is a technique for removing them with a minimum risk of further damage.

First loop a long piece of string round the hook. Press down on the shank of the hook, so it lies flat along the skin. Hold

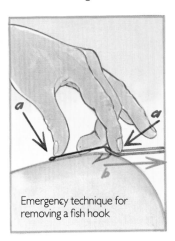

Emergency technique for removing a fish hook

it down as you gradually tighten the string.

Now give a sharp pull, parallel with the skin, and the hook will come straight out through the hole it made as it entered.

Clean and dress the wound, and if there is any sign of infection within the next few days get medical attention.

Food Poisoning see POISONING, page 85.

Foreign Bodies

Foreign bodies may become lodged in the eyes, ears, or nose. They may be swallowed or inhaled, also. Children are particularly prone to such hazards.

The Eye: small foreign bodies are often cleared by the normal reflex action of blinking. If the pain persists, **do not** rub the eye, as this would scratch the cornea.

If the irritant cannot be seen, or is lying on or embedded in the surface of the eyeball, **do not** attempt first aid.

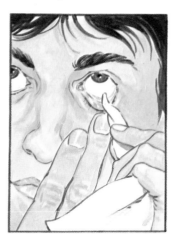

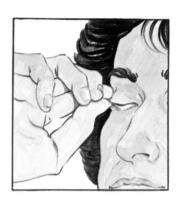

Cover the eye with a clean dressing, and obtain immediate medical attention at hospital.

Often the foreign body will be low down in the eye, resting against the lower lid. Pull down the lower lid, and carefully remove the irritant with the corner of a clean handkerchief, or a swab of damp cotton wool.

If the irritant is under the *upper* eyelid, ask the casualty to look down, then gently pull the eyelid out and down over the lower eyelid. The eyelashes of the lower lid will usually dislodge the object. If this does not work, the casualty should blink the eye repeatedly under water, either using an eyebath or submerging the whole face in a basin of water.

If these measures are unsuccessful, get medical attention.

The Ears and Nose: children often poke beads, plasticine, etc. into their ears or nostrils. There is no immediate risk, but **do not** attempt to remove the object yourself, as you may push it further in. Take the child to the doctor or hospital.

Insects occasionally find their way into an ear, unlikely as this sounds. They can be floated out with luke warm water or olive oil. Simply tilt the head to the opposite side, gently pull the earlobe backwards and insert a few drops of water or olive oil. Keep the head tilted for a few minutes, then allow the water or olive oil to run out with the insect. No further treatment will be necessary unless it was a stinging insect, in which case, get medical attention.

Inhaled Foreign Bodies: see CHOKING, page 68.

Swallowed Objects: often a "swallowed" object is merely lodged in the back of the throat. If this is the case, the casualty should lean over the back of a chair, head down lower than his chest, while you deliver a series of sharp thumps between his shoulder blades. This should be quite sufficient to dislodge the irritant.

If an object has been swallowed, find out quickly what it was. If it was something smooth, like a coin or a stone, it will almost certainly be eliminated naturally within a few days. Tell the doctor anyway.

If the object was sharp or jagged, **do not** attempt any first aid – get the casualty to hospital **as fast as possible**.

Fractures see BROKEN BONES AND DISLOCATION, page 61.

Frostbite

Frostbite occurs when extreme cold causes tiny blood vessels in the skin to become narrowed, cutting off the blood supply to extremities like the nose, fingers, and toes.

The first symptom is numbness; the affected parts become white and the power of movement is lost. If prolonged, this can lead to gangrene of the frostbitten parts. Remove constrictive items such as rings, watches, gloves and shoes. **Do not** rub the affected part, or apply direct heat. Get the casualty into a warm sheltered place and give him warm drinks, allowing him to warm through gradually and naturally. Cover the affected parts with warm blankets; tuck frostbitten hands under the armpits. As the frozen parts begin to thaw, they will be extremely painful. Get qualified medical treatment as soon as possible, as there is a risk of subsequent damage.
□See also EXPOSURE.

Gassing see CARBON MON-OXIDE POISONING, page 33.

Hangover

A hangover is the result of an intake of too much alcohol. The body is dehydrated, due to excessive water loss in the urine. The stomach may be raw, causing queaziness. The headache results from the dehydration, and the small amounts of chemicals present in certain alcoholic drinks such as brandy, sherry, or red wine.

Drink large quantities of water or milk to replace body fluid. *Do not* take aspirin for the headache; even the soluble form will only make stomach inflammation worse. Just keep drinking water or milk, and wear dark glasses or an eyeshade if the eyes are painful.

Head Injuries and Concussion

Minor head injuries, such as cuts, scrapes, and bruises, can be treated at home. But if the casualty has been knocked out, even for a moment, a doctor's advice should be sought. More serious injuries to the head can be very dangerous, and always need medical advice and treatment. These are of two types, involving either skull fractures, or injury to the brain.

Concussion is the most common of these accidents. It occurs after a solid blow on the head, or sometimes after a fall onto rigidly extended legs, where the shock is carried directly up the spine to the brain. The violent movement literally "rattles" the brain in the skull, causing stupor or unconsciousness. This is the almost immediate effect of the injury, and is accompanied by paleness, clammy skin, and shallow breathing. As the casualty recovers, he may vomit. There is usually loss of memory of events just before and just after the accident.

Concussion always needs urgent medical attention. First aid measures are as for UNCONSCIOUSNESS (page 41), plus treatment for any visible injuries.

Sometimes a blow on the head causes the more serious condition of brain compression, where there is pressure on the brain caused by a skull fracture, or bleeding within the skull. It sometimes follows concussion.

Symptoms of brain compression differ from concussion. The casualty may sometimes have a convulsion. Typically, breathing is noisy, and the face flushed rather than pale.

The most characteristic symptom is that the pupils of the eyes appear abnormal. They may be larger than usual, or of unequal size. The casualty may remain conscious for a while before slipping into a coma.

This is an extremely serious condition, and medical aid must be obtained urgently. While waiting for medical aid to arrive, take all precautions to maintain the casualty's breathing (see UNCONSCIOUSNESS, page 41).

First aid for a fractured skull depends very much on the site and type of injury. Sometimes a fracture is detectable by finding blood or yellowish fluid running from the ear or nose after a blow on the head or an accident which has severely shaken the head. In a heavy blow to the face, the cheekbones or jaw may be broken. These injuries are less serious, provided there is no obstruction to breathing.

Obstructed breathing is the greatest hazard in any severe head injury. While unconscious, the casualty cannot cough and clear blood or vomit from the airways.

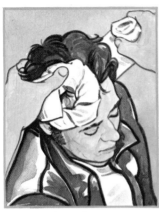

A ring bandage will prevent direct pressure over wound

After checking that mouth and throat are not obstructed, and that the casualty is breathing properly, turn him into the RECOVERY POSITION (page 41), and check frequently that breathing is being maintained. Be ready to start ARTIFICIAL RESPIRATION (page 44) at any time.

If the casualty has only moderate injuries to face or jaw, he can sit up, leaning forward to prevent blood draining back into the throat.

Obtain medical aid urgently.

Heart Attack

Blockage or narrowing of blood vessels supplying the heart muscle causes acute chest pain, often spreading through the left shoulder and down the left arm. It is usually accompanied by breathlessness and weakness. The casualty's heart may beat erratically.

An attack caused by narrowed blood vessels is called *angina pectoris*. This may affect a person periodically over many years, and most people with angina carry with them special tablets which dissolve under the tongue and relieve the pain within a few minutes.

Angina pectoris attacks are brought on by exertion or excitement, and usually clear when the patient sits or lies down and rests. Help the patient to take any "heart tablets" he may be carrying, and get him to hospital as soon as possible.

A true heart attack, or coronary thrombosis, is brought on by blockage of a blood vessel. It may come on slowly, with a gradual feeling of tiredness and heaviness in the left shoulder, or with dramatic suddenness, as though the chest were gripped in a vice.

Lay the casualty down with head and shoulders supported on a couple of pillows, so that he is half-sitting. Loosen any restrictive clothing, and send for medical aid immediately.

ARTIFICIAL RESPIRATION (page 44) will be necessary if breathing fails. HEART MASSAGE (page 46) may also be necessary, but **only** if you are certain the heart has stopped.

Heat Stroke

Overexertion in hot weather or exposure to unaccustomed tropical climates can cause heat exhaustion. This condition comes on gradually, and is a form of shock due to excessive losses of salt and water. This can happen as a result of sweating or severe diarrhoea which is common in newcomers to hot climates.

Early symptoms are muscle cramps, rapid pulse and breathing, and a pale, clammy skin. This state can continue for several days, and is eventually followed by fainting.

The casualty must rest in a cool place, and drink large amounts of cool water or fruit juice, to which has been added 1/2 teaspoonful of table salt per 600 ml (1 pint).

In heat exhaustion, the body maintains a fairly normal temperature, by copious sweating. If the body's temperature regulation system fails because of prolonged heat or illness, the more dangerous heat stroke can occur quite suddenly.

The casualty appears flushed and restless, and the pulse is very strong. Breathing is deep and noisy, and the skin is burning hot.

The aim of first aid is to get the body temperature down rapidly, before the casualty loses consciousness and lapses into a coma.

Remove the casualty's clothes, and sponge him all over with cool water (**do not** use ice). Wrap him in wet sheets, and turn him into the RECOVERY POSITION (page 41).

Fan the casualty to produce a current of cooling air.

When the casualty begins to recover, cover him with dry sheets, and get medical attention as soon as possible. Be prepared to repeat the temperature reducing measures if the casualty becomes distressed again.

Hernia

Hernia or rupture is a tear in the sheets of muscles covering the abdomen, allowing some of the internal organs to bulge through. There is a weak point in the groin, where most hernias occur, although they may also appear at the site of an old operation scar, or at the navel. Hernias are usually caused by severe exertion, such as lifting a very heavy object.

The condition is usually painless at first, but may later be uncomfortable and vomiting may occur. Hernias are not normally dangerous, provided they receive prompt medical treatment.

Lay the casualty down, with head and shoulders supported on cushions, and the knees raised to reduce tension on the abdominal muscles. This should relieve the pain and allow the casualty to get to a doctor. **Do not** attempt to press back the bulge of the hernia. If the hernia is causing severe pain, get medical attention before allowing the casualty to move.

Holiday Problems

Any of the accidents discussed in this book can spoil a holiday, but there are more specific holiday problems, some of which can be avoided by forethought. If going abroad, check with your travel agent *and* the doctor several weeks before to see what vaccinations are recommended for the countries you are visiting. The requirements vary from year to year, and even if you have previously had the appropriate "shots", you may need a booster. If you are holidaying in any country where there is a risk of contracting malaria ask your doctor for a course of tablets.

Jellyfish Stings: jellyfish stings are very painful but not usually serious. The only common dangerous type is the Portuguese Man-of-War, which has a blue or lavender coloured bladder floating on the surface like an inflated plastic bag. Keep well clear of its tentacles.

Do not rub off the sting – saturate in alcohol (methylated spirit, gin or whisky), then when it shrivels it can be wiped off.

For mild jellyfish stings, apply calamine cream or lotion, or antihistamine cream if there is much redness and swelling. For a severe sting, get medical help quickly. (See also BITES AND STINGS, page 60.)

Sea urchins: spikey urchins are found in most warm seas, over rocks. Their spines are sharp and brittle, breaking off beneath the skin when trodden on – or when sat on. Because they are so brittle, they must be pulled out *straight*.

Get medical help if there are many spikes left beneath the skin. Single spines are painful, but gradually dissolve and disappear without further attention.

Holiday diarrhoea: mild cases of diarrhoea can be treated with kaolin and morphine mixture, but in some foreign countries, more serious diarrhoea is often a problem.

In many countries, antibiotics can be bought freely, and the doctor or pharmacist will recommend one suitable for your problem. Always take the whole course of antibiotic, otherwise the condition may return. Drink plenty of fluids, adding ½ teaspoonful of table salt to each 600 ml (1 pint) of water, or take salt tablets. If holiday diarrhoea does not respond to treatment within 2–3 days, consult a doctor.

Local illnesses: if you are travelling abroad there are many "local illnesses" to which your body is not accustomed, and which therefore pose a threat. Some are minor; some very serious. Take no chances with *any* illness which does not clear up quickly. Get local medical treatment or, if you feel ill shortly after returning from holiday, consult your own doctor and tell him where you have been.

Take with you:
Travel sickness pills
Soluble Aspirin BP and Junior
  Aspirin
Pack of assorted dressings
Insect repellent and Calamine
  lotion
Water tablets (if visiting country
  where water is unsafe)
Salt tablets (if visiting country
  where climate is very hot).
☐See also HEAT STROKE,
INSECT BITES, and SNAKE BITES.

Hysteria

An hysterical attack sometimes follows an emotional upset, or severe stress. It can resemble an epileptic fit, but has an important difference, in that the casualty remains completely conscious throughout. The hysteria is intended for the benefit of the onlookers, to gain their sympathy, and is a variant of the temper tantrums so common in young children. It should *not* be dismissed as a form of malingering, however; it is a psychological reaction to stress, and may be completely involuntary in an excitable or "nervous" person.

In an hysterical attack, the casualty may shout, scream, roll on the ground, go rigid, or hold the breath. Unlike epilepsy, he will not injure himself and will always retain sufficient awareness to be conscious of what is going on around him.

Do not slap an hysterical person to "bring him around". This merely gives him the attention he craves. Clear away *all* onlookers, to deny him an audience. Calm the casualty by speaking in a firm, "no-nonsense" voice, and try to distract him, e.g., by giving him a warm drink.

When he appears calmer, get him to a doctor, in case further treatment is necessary.

Insect Bites and Stings

Insect stings, such as those caused by wasps and bees, are immediately painful. Sometimes the sting remains in the wound, looking like a small splinter. This must be removed with tweezers. Grip the sting close to where it has entered the skin. **Do not** grip the far end of the sting, as this may pump more venom into the wound.

If the sting is very short, dislodge it with a needle which has been passed through a flame to sterilise it, and then allowed to cool.

Relieve pain and itching from stings or bites with antihistamine cream, which can be bought at any chemist. If this is not available, sponge the bite or sting with a solution of bicarbonate of soda, or apply a cold compress.

If pain and inflammation get worse over the next few days, see a doctor, as the wound is probably infected.

Bites or stings in the mouth can be dangerous, as the swelling may obstruct breathing. Rinse the mouth with a solution of bicarbonate of soda or suck ice

Grip sting close to where it entered the skin

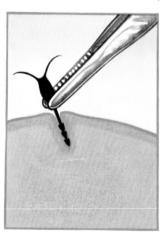

cubes to minimise swelling, and obtain emergency medical treatment.

Very rarely, the whole system reacts violently after an insect sting or bite. The casualty becomes pale and shocked, and may lose consciousness rapidly. Turn him into the RECOVERY POSITION (page 41) and obtain medical treatment as fast as possible. This is a serious emergency. While waiting for help to arrive, watch the casualty to make sure breathing is not affected (see BREATHING PROBLEMS, page 42).

Lightning

Injuries caused by lightning are the same as those caused by contact with high-tension electricity cables. The casualty may be killed immediately, or merely stunned. Deep internal burning may occur. Treat any obvious external burns, call for medical aid urgently, and give ARTIFICIAL RESPIRATION (page 44) if breathing is affected. □See also BREATHING PROBLEMS, and BURNS.

Migraine

Migraine is a form of severe headache often accompanied by sickness and blurred or distorted vision. It usually affects only one side of the head. The causes are not understood, but it is sometimes associated with emotional problems, and is also suspected of being caused sometimes by a food allergy.

Attacks can last for several hours, and recur at irregular intervals. During a migraine attack, rest in a darkened room. Special drugs may have been prescribed; otherwise aspirin or strong coffee sometimes provide relief.

Miscarriage

Following an illness, a pregnant woman may miscarry. Miscarriage is also the body's natural way of aborting a foetus which is not developing properly. Sometimes it occurs because of some weakness or damage to the neck of the womb.

A miscarriage is more likely during the early stages of the pregnancy. Bleeding from the vagina may be very slight, or may be heavy and accompanied by period-like pains. *Any* such bleeding or pain must be treated as a threatened miscarriage. Call the doctor **immediately**. While waiting for medical help to arrive, get the casualty to lie down and remain as still as possible. An *external* sanitary towel will help with the bleeding.

Mouth Injuries

Lip or cheek injury: injuries due to accidental self-inflicted bites bleed copiously. Bleeding can be stopped by covering the injury with a clean gauze dressing, and pinching the injured area firmly between finger and thumb – applying pressure on both sides. Bleeding will usually stop within a few minutes. If not, get medical attention.
Bitten tongue: the tongue should be extended, then

gripped firmly with a clean dry cloth. Pull the tongue out gently but firmly, without causing discomfort. This constricts blood vessels at the base of the tongue, and should stop the bleeding within 10 minutes. If not, get medical assistance.

Bleeding from the teeth: bleeding from a tooth socket is seldom serious, and can usually be checked by biting firmly into a wad of clean, rolled cloth. Keep up the pressure for 20 minutes, then remove the cloth very gently so as not to disturb the blood clot. Repeat if necessary, and get medical assistance if bleeding cannot be stopped.

Serious mouth injuries: see HEAD INJURIES, page 78, for damage to face and jaw.

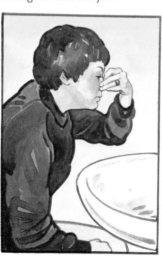

For nosebleeds, tilt head slightly down and pinch lower nostrils between finger and thumb for at least 10 minutes, breathing through mouth. Release nostrils slowly

Nosebleeds

A nosebleed may follow a knock on the nose, or may happen spontaneously, when a small blood vessel in the nose ruptures.

Sit the casualty down, leaning well forward, get him to pinch the soft lower part of his nose firmly between finger and thumb, and breathe through his mouth. Keep the nostrils pinched shut for at least 10 minutes, then release them slowly. If the nose continues to bleed, pinch the nostrils shut once more. If the bleeding cannot be stopped in this way, get the casualty to hospital, still pinching his nostrils together.

Once bleeding has stopped, the casualty should not blow his nose for several hours.

Penetrating Wounds

A puncture or stab through the skin leaves a deceptively small hole. The wound beneath may be very deep, and the object which caused the wound may have been dirty. Contamination could be carried deep within the wound, and infection is probable.

For this reason, make no attempt to check the bleeding, which carries dirt *out* of the wound. When the bleeding stops naturally, apply a dressing and get the casualty to a doctor, unless the wound is small and shallow, in which case treat as for CUTS AND GRAZES (page 70). If in any doubt, get medical attention, as there is a risk of tetanus or other infections from a deep wound, especially if it is dirty.

Chest injuries: deep wounds to the chest may puncture the lungs, and are very serious. See chest injuries under BROKEN BONES AND DISLOCATIONS, (page 64).

Poisoning

Two major groups of chemicals cause poisoning when taken by mouth. These are:

1. Poisons acting directly on the mouth, throat, stomach, and the rest of the digestive system. Symptoms caused by absorption into the system may occur later. Typical of these poisons are contaminated or rotten food, and some poisonous plants.

Some of these poisons are corrosive, causing immediate burning and pain. Examples are: bleach, petrol, disinfectants, strong acids, and alkalis like caustic soda (sometimes included in oven cleaner).

2. Other poisons act on the nervous system after absorption into the body. Their effects are therefore delayed, and because immediate first aid may not be undertaken, they are doubly dangerous. Once symptoms appear, it is usually too late to remove the poison from the system by inducing vomiting. Among these poisons are aspirin and other pain-killing drugs, sleeping tablets, and poisonous toadstools.

Other less common forms of poisoning are caused by inhaling fumes, see CARBON MONOXIDE POISONING (page 33), DRUGS AND ALCOHOL (page 72), and accidental or intentional injection of a chemical through the skin. Certain industrial and garden chemicals, such as insecticides, can be absorbed directly through the skin in sufficient quantity to cause poisoning.

If you suspect that someone has taken poison by mouth, act very rapidly.

While the casualty is conscious, ask what poison they may have taken. If the casualty knows he has taken a corrosive poison, or if the mouth and lips are sore or blistered, give him large quantities of water or milk to dilute the poison. Wipe away poison from around the mouth. **Do not** try to make the casualty vomit. Arrange transport to hospital by car as fast as possible and have someone telephone the hospital to tell them the casualty is on the way.

If you are sure that the poison was non-corrosive, and the casualty is conscious, make him vomit by pushing two fingers right down the back of his throat. Protect your fingers from bites by jamming a rolled-up handkerchief in the corner of the casualty's mouth. Let the casualty drink plenty of water between each bout of induced vomiting, to flush out the poison. Watch carefully to make sure that no vomit is inhaled. Remove the casualty to hospital quickly. **Do not** induce vomiting if the casualty is unconscious.

Unconscious casualties should

be turned into the RECOVERY POSITION (page 41). Call for emergency medical assistance, and be prepared to give ARTIFICIAL RESPIRATION (page 44) if breathing stops.

Do not attempt to give liquids to an unconscious casualty.

In all cases, try to save some of the poison, vomited material, or medicine containers to help the hospital identify the substance.

Agricultural chemicals and garden pesticides: these substances are powerful nerve poisons, and can cause a wide range of symptoms, including twitching muscles and convulsions. Sometimes symptoms occur several hours after handling or using pesticides. These require immediate medical attention, as they could be the forerunners of serious poisoning.

Casualties must rest completely while awaiting medical aid. Strip off clothing splashed with chemicals, and wash the body thoroughly. If a pesticide has been taken by mouth give large quantities of water to drink.

Sleeping tablets and tranquillisers: these drugs affect breathing, and ARTIFICIAL RESPIRATION (page 44) and HEART MASSAGE (page 46) may be necessary while waiting for medical assistance.

Attempted suicide: a person who has attempted suicide by overdosing with medicines should be made to vomit, as these substances are unlikely to

be corrosive. ARTIFICIAL RESPIRATION may be necessary.

If the attempted suicide was by drinking disinfectant or bleach (usually detectable by smelling the breath) treat by giving copious drinks of water or milk. **Do not** induce vomiting.

Get urgent medical assistance in any attempted suicide.

Rashes

A rash is local inflammation of the skin, caused by any of a variety of factors. Allergic reactions to something in contact with the skin can cause rashes, as can drugs and infections such as measles and scarlet fever.

Treat the rash with calamine cream or lotion, or with an antihistamine cream, and seek medical attention for any underlying illness.

Shock see page 50.

Snake Bites

Snake bites are rare in Britain, and the adder is the only one of our native snakes that is poisonous. Even the adder is not nearly as poisonous as many foreign snakes, and deaths are extremely rare. The non-poisonous grass snake and smooth snake occasionally bite if provoked. Slow worms, often mistaken for snakes, are quite harmless.

Shock is the worst risk in snakebite, and causes more problems than the bite itself (see SHOCK, page 50). An Adder bite causes immediate sharp

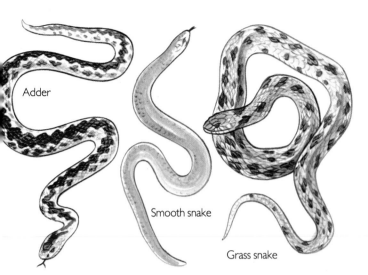

Adder

Smooth snake

Grass snake

pain, followed by swelling around the bite. Other more serious symptoms are vomiting, sweating, and faintness, but these are quite rare.

Do not cut the wound open to let out the venom. **Do not** apply a tourniquet. Calm and reassure the casualty, and keep him still to reduce circulation of the venom. Wash the wound with soapy water and cover it with a dry, sterile dressing. Give aspirin or paracetamol to reduce the pain.

Immobilise bitten limbs, by tying ankles loosely together, or putting the arm in a sling (see BANDAGING AND WOUND DRESSING, page 58).

Get the casualty to hospital as quickly as possible. Be on guard for any deterioration in breathing (see BREATHING PROBLEMS, page 42).

If the snake has been caught or killed, take it to hospital to aid in identification of the poison.

Splinters and Thorns

Splinters and thorns cause only minor wounds, but these can be extremely painful and can become infected, if the object causing the wound was dirty.

Sometimes a splinter or thorn can be gripped between clean finger nails, or by tweezers, and pulled straight out along the direction in which it penetrated the skin.

If a splinter or thorn lies below the skin surface, either leave it to work its way out naturally over the course of a few weeks, or prise it out carefully, using a needle tip, sterilised in a flame then allowed to cool,

If the splinter has gone straight in, it is sometimes possible to spike it sideways with the needle tip, and draw it out far enough to grip with tweezers.

Splinters or thorns lying sideways just beneath the skin can be removed by pricking gently with the sterilised needle until the skin above the object has been opened. The end of the splinter can then be hooked out and gripped with tweezers.

Wounds caused by splinters and thorns which subsequently become infected, or any wound caused by metal or glass splinters, need medical attention.

Splints

Splints are rigid supports, bound to a broken arm or leg to immobilise the limb while a casualty is being transported to hospital.

Usually, splinting is unnecessary in domestic accidents, as the doctor or ambulance personnel will quickly arrange to transport the casualty to hospital, so the need for first aid is minimised. If, however, an accident takes place in an inaccessible area, proper immobilisation is essential.

The requirements for a splint are simple:
1. It must be rigid and long enough to be fastened securely above and below the break.
2. It must be adequately padded, so that it is comfortable when fitted along the limb.
Emergency splints can be improvised from any suitable material, such as pieces of wood, walking sticks, broom handles or tightly rolled newspapers.
□ See also BROKEN BONES AND DISLOCATIONS

Stab Wounds see
PENETRATING WOUNDS, page 84.

Strokes

A stroke is caused by bleeding or blockage (thrombosis) of a blood vessel in the brain, which produces widely varying symptoms. In a very mild stroke, there may be a severe headache, minor clumsiness affecting the arm or leg on one side of the body, or just a drooping eyelid.

In more serious strokes, there may be obvious paralysis, slurred speech, or complete collapse. Get the casualty to bed immediately and call the doctor. There are no specific first aid measures you can take, other than making the casualty comfortable and reassuring him while awaiting medical help, and by keeping him breathing properly.

If the casualty is semi-conscious or unconscious, place him in the RECOVERY POSITION (page 41).

Strains and Sprains

A strain is damage to a muscle, usually caused by overstretching it in a sudden jerk or fall. Sometimes muscle fibres are torn. There is sharp muscular pain, and perhaps swelling.
Minor strains are treated by resting the damaged muscle. A cold compress reduces later swelling, and firm binding with a crêpe bandage provides support. Severe strains need medical treatment, and must be immobilised while transporting the casualty to hospital.
A sprain is quite different, affecting only the joint. It

resembles a dislocation, except that joint damage is limited to tearing of the tendons which hold the joint together.

Sprains are very painful, and the casualty must immediately take all the weight off the damaged limb and support it in a comfortable position. Apply cold compresses to the joint to reduce later swelling, then bandage firmly but lightly with a crêpe bandage, to provide support.

Shoes or boots may be left on to provide extra support for sprained ankles.

Get medical attention if pain and swelling persist.
☐See also BROKEN BONES AND DISLOCATION

Sunburn

The effects of excessive sun on unprotected skin are well known: first reddening, then soreness and sometimes blistering.

Treat reddened and tender skin with calamine lotion or cream. Blistering on small areas, such as lips or nose, can be treated with antihistamine cream. If blistering covers large areas of skin, or if the burned person is shivering, consult a doctor.
☐See also HEAT STROKE

Travel Sickness

Travel sickness (sea sickness, motion sickness) is caused by disturbance of the organs of balance, due to unaccustomed or extreme movements of the body.

Take a proprietary travel sickness remedy before journeys, if you anticipate any problem. **Do not** give tablets containing *hyoscine* to young children. Always follow the dosage properly.

Minimise the risk of sickness by taking sensible precautions. Take a light meal before travelling; *do not* read or lie down while in motion. Try to arrange good ventilation, or direct a light breeze on to your face.

If you do experience travel sickness, the unpleasant symptoms should clear up within an hour of completing your journey.

Unconsciousness see page 41

Vomiting

Vomiting is a symptom of some other problem. It can be associated with fainting, shock, poisoning, or an infectious disease, and is often the body's way of disposing of materials which irritate the stomach. Vomiting is tiring and very uncomfortable, leaving the stomach muscles sore and aching. The stomach acids in vomit can burn the mouth and throat, leaving an unpleasant sour taste.

Rinse the mouth thoroughly after vomiting, and sip small amounts of tepid water to replace body fluids without provoking further vomiting attacks. Report the incident to the doctor if it happens again, or if blood appears in the vomit.

4: First Aid Kits

The Home Medicine Chest

You can buy a complete first aid kit from larger chemists' shops, but it is often less expensive to assemble your own. If you decide on the latter course, here is a list of useful items for first aid *and* home treatment. As they are used, replace them with fresh supplies.

Perforated film (non-stick) dressings; small, medium and large

Triangular bandages for slings

Rolled gauze bandages; assorted sizes

Adhesive plasters; assorted sizes

Adhesive plaster strip, 1 roll, for attaching dressing and securing bandages

Sterile cotton wool

Safety pins; assorted sizes

Scissors; preferably blunt-tipped

Crêpe bandages, for sprains and strains

Aspirin "Soluble" tablets BP, or paracetamol tablets BP

Calamine cream or lotion

Antihistamine cream

Disinfectant; medicinal quality

Tweezers; with fine points

Travel sickness tablets

Medical thermometer

Cotton wool buds

Kaolin and morphine mixture, to relieve diarrhoea.

Sodium bicarbonate powder

Never keep left-over medicines or pills prescribed by your doctor for a specific purpose. Dispose of them by flushing them down the lavatory. **Never** give them to anyone other than the person for whom they were prescribed.
Always keep all medicines, tablets and pills well out of reach of young children and preferably locked away.

How to use a thermometer

A medical thermometer is a useful item to keep in the household medicine chest.
When not in use, keep it in its protective case. Before use, it must be rinsed in cold water, and wiped with clean cotton

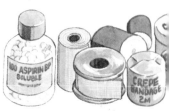

wool. Grip the stem of the thermometer firmly, and shake down the thread of mercury with a series of sharp flicks. The mercury thread should rest near the bottom end of the marked scale.

Now place the bulb end of the thermometer under the tongue, and close the lips around it – without gripping the thermometer in the teeth. Keep it in place for 2 minutes precisely.

Remove the thermometer and read off the temperature – that is, the highest point to which the mercury has risen on the scale. Normal body temperature falls between 36°–37°C (Centigrade or Celsius) or 97°–99°F (Farenheit). Temperatures above this range are usually due to infections. Lower temperatures occur after infection has passed, in shock, fainting, and in hypothermia.

Bear in mind that temperatures vary at different times of day.

Shake down the mercury, and clean the thermometer in a solution of antiseptic and cold water. Wipe it dry with a swab of cotton wool and return it to the storage case.

In babies, temperature can be taken under the armpit. Dry the skin and the thermometer, place the bulb under the baby's arm, then hold the arm folded across the chest for 2 minutes. Check temperature as before. This method is not always reliable, and the procedure may need to be repeated.

Do not attempt to take the temperature by inserting a thermometer into the back passage. This is very dangerous unless special training has been given.

Do not attempt to take the temperature of an unconscious casualty.

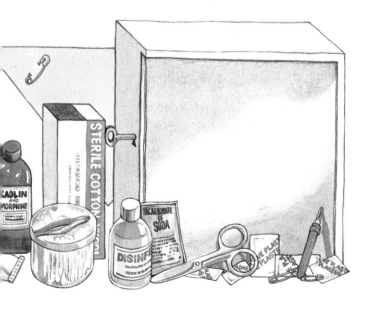

First Aid Kit for the Motorist

A number of prepacked First Aid kits are available specially designed to be carried in the car. The contents vary, but all such kits must be packed in a strong container which will not spill the contents out in the glove box or parcel shelf. In addition to the First Aid kit, make sure you have available in the car other items which may be useful in an emergency, such as a torch, fire extinguisher (of the proper type for use in the car) and red warning triangles, to warn oncoming traffic of a breakdown or accident.

A good basic First Aid kit will contain:

Perforated film (non-stick) dressing; large

Rolled crêpe bandages; wide

Adhesive plasters; assorted sizes

Adhesive plaster strip; 1 roll. For attaching dressings and securing bandages

Sterile cotton wool

Triangular bandages; for use as a sling

Medicated tissues; pre-soaked in germicide

Antiseptic cream (there will be no opportunity to dilute ordinary antiseptic)

Scissors; preferably blunt-tipped

Tweezers, with fine points

Safety pins; assorted sizes

Antihistamine cream

Aspirin "Soluble" tablets BP, or paracetamol tablets BP

Rescue blanket, of metalised plastic. Available from camping equipment suppliers. Folds up very small, but unfolds to a size large enough to wrap over the whole body. Used to keep casualty warm – important in shock or exposure.

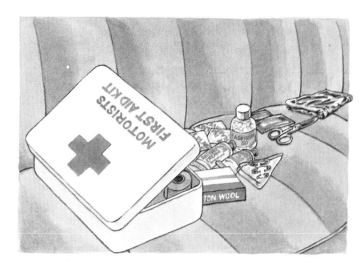

Emergency Telephone List

Doctor

Surgery Address

Telephone

Surgery Hours   Night Service

Hospital for emergencies

Address

Telephone

Dentist

Surgery Address

Telephone

Surgery Hours

Local Gas Emergency Service: telephone

FIRE
POLICE   Dial 999 and ask operator for
AMBULANCE   the relevant emergency service(s)

Nearest Taxi Services: telephone

Persons to contact in emergency

Name

Address

Telephone   Business Telephone

Name

Address

Telephone   Business Telephone

Index